# FUNDAMENTALS OF
# English
# Grammar

## FIFTH EDITION
## VOLUME B

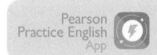

Pearson
Practice English
App

## Betty S. Azar
## Stacy A. Hagen

**Fundamentals of English Grammar, Fifth Edition**
**with Pearson Practice English App**
**Volume B**

Azar Associates: Sue Van Etten, Manager

Pearson Education, 221 River Street, Hoboken, NJ 07030

**Staff credits:** The people who made up the *Fundamentals of English Grammar Fifth Edition* team, representing content development, design, multimedia, project management, publishing, and rights management, are Pietro Alongi, Sheila Ameri, Jennifer Castro, Tracey Cataldo, Dave Dickey, Gina DiLillo, Warren Fischbach, Sarah Henrich, Niki Lee, Stefan Machura, Amy McCormick, Robert Ruvo, Katarzyna Starzynska-Kosciuszko, Paula Van Ells, Joseph Vella, and Marcin Wozniak.

Contributing Editors: Barbara Lyons, Janice L. Baillie
Text composition: Aptara

Disclaimer: This work is produced by Pearson Education and is not endorsed by any trademark owner referenced in this publication.

**Library of Congress Cataloging-in-Publication Data**

A catalog record for the print edition is available from the Library of Congress.

Printed in the United States of America
ISBN 13: 978-0-13-511657-9
ISBN 10: 0-13-511657-0

51 2023

*To*
*Shelley Hartle and Sue Van Etten*
B.S.A.


*To the students and teachers at*
*Edmonds Community College,*
*from whom I learned so much*
S.A.H.

# Contents

# Preface to the Fifth Edition

*Fundamentals of English Grammar* is an intermediate skills text for English language learners. It functions principally as a classroom teaching text but also serves as a comprehensive reference for students and teachers.

Using a time-tested approach that has helped millions of students around the world, *Fundamentals of English Grammar* blends direct grammar instruction with carefully sequenced practice to develop speaking, writing, listening, and reading skills. Grammar is not a mere collection of rules; rather, it is presented as a framework for organizing English. Students have a natural, logical way to help make sense of the language they see and hear.

This edition has been extensively revised to keep pace with advances in theory and practice, particularly from cognitive science. We are excited to introduce important new features and updates.

- **A pretest at the start of each chapter** allows learners to assess what they already know and orient themselves to the chapter material. Research indicates that taking a pretest may enhance learning even if a student gets every answer wrong.
- **Practice, spaced out over time**, helps students learn better. Numerous exercises have been added to provide more incremental practice.
- **New charts and exercises show patterns** to help learners make sense of the information. This reflects research showing that the adult brain is wired to look for patterns.
- **Meaning-based practice** is introduced at the sentence level. Students do not have to wait for longer passages to work with meaning, as is the case with many textbooks.
- **Frequent oral exercises** encourage students to speak more naturally and fluidly, in other words, with more automaticity—an important marker of fluency.
- **Step-by-step writing activities** promote written fluency. All end-of-chapter tasks include writing tips and editing checklists.
- **A wide range of contextualized exercises,** with an emphasis on life-skills vocabulary, encourages authentic language use.
- **Updated grammar charts** based on corpus research reflect current usage and highlight the differences between written and spoken English in formal and informal contexts.
- The **BlackBookBlog,** new to this edition, focuses on student success, cultural differences, and life-skills strategies.
- **End-of-chapter Learning Checks** help students assess their learning.

Now more than ever, teachers will find an extensive range of presentations, activities, and tasks to meet the specific needs of their classes.

Components of *Fundamentals of English Grammar,* Fifth Edition

- **Online Resources**
  - For the teacher: **Teacher's Guide** and front-of-classroom **PowerPoint** presentations
  - For the student: A Pearson Practice English **App** (with diagnostic tests, end-of-chapter Learning Checks, review tests, Student Book audio, and guided **PowerPoint** videos)
- A comprehensive **Workbook** that consists of self-study exercises for independent work
- A **Teacher's Guide** that features step-by-step teaching instructions for each chart, notes on key grammar structures, vocabulary lists, and expansion activities
- A revised **Test Bank** with quizzes, chapter tests, and mid-term and final exams
- A **Chartbook,** a reference book that consists of only the grammar charts

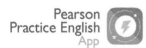

- Diagnostic tests
- End-of-chapter Learning Checks
- Review tests
- Student Book audio
- Guided PowerPoint videos

The Azar-Hagen Grammar Series consists of

- *Understanding and Using English Grammar* (blue cover), for upper-level students.
- *Fundamentals of English Grammar* (black cover), for mid-level students.
- *Basic English Gramm*ar (red cover), for lower or beginning levels.

# Acknowledgments

We are indebted to the reviewers and other outstanding teachers who contributed to this edition by giving us extensive feedback on the Fourth edition and helping us shape the new Fifth edition.

In particular, we would like to thank Tammy Adams, University of Missouri-Kansas City; Maureen S. Andrade, Utah Valley University; Dorothy Avondstondt, Miami Dade College; Judith Campbell, University of Montreal; Shirlaine B. Castellino, Spring International Language Center, CO; Holly Cin, Houston Community College; Eileen M. Cotter, Montgomery College, MD; Yecsenia Delgado, Monrovia Adult School, CA; Andrew Donlan, International Language Institute, Washington, D.C.; Gillian L. Durham, Tidewater Community College; Jill M. Fox, University of Nebraska; Frank Grandits, City College of San Francisco; William Hennessey IV, Florida International University; Clay Hindman, Sierra Community College; Zoe Isaacson, Queens College; Barbara Jaccarino, Brooklyn College; Sharla Jones, San Antonio College; Balynda Kelly Foster, Spring International Language Center, CO; Noga Laor, Long Island University; Ann Larios, Queens College; Sara Miller, Queens College; June Ohrnberger, Suffolk County Community College, NY; Deniz Ozgorgulu, Bogazici University, Turkey; Jan Peterson, Edmonds Community College; Miriam Pollack, Grossmont College; Ray Schiel, College of English Language, Santa Monica, CA; Malek Shawareb, Houston Community College; Carol Siegel, Community College of Baltimore County; Elizabeth Marie Van Amerongen, Community College of Baltimore County; Laura Vance, Spring International Language Center, CO; Melissa Villamil, Houston Community College; Daniela C. Wagner-Loera, University of Maryland, College Park; Summer Webb, University of Colorado-Boulder; Kirsten Windahl, Cuyahoga Community College; Katarina Zorkic, Rosemead College of English.

We thank the teachers of the focus group at Edmonds Community College for their invaluable feedback: Linda Carlson, Jan Peterson, Patrick Rolland, Ruth Voetmann, and Kelly Roberts Weibel.

We once again had a stellar management and editorial team every step of the way. Product Manager Amy McCormick oversaw the project with insight and vision. We were fortunate to once again have Senior Content Producer Robert Ruvo, who deftly juggled the many components of this revision and kept us on track. Barbara Lyons, our development editor, shaped the charts, exercises, and layout with precision and care. Janice Baillie, our production editor, lent her eagle eye to every detail on every page. We are grateful as always to Sue Van Etten for her expert business management of Azar Associates.

We'd also like to thank our talented supplement writers: Geneva Tesh, Houston Community College, for the revised Workbook, MyEnglishLab, and PowerPoint material; Kelly Roberts Weibel, Edmonds Community College, for the updated Test Bank, and Ruth Voetmann, Edmonds Community College, for the reworked Teacher's Guide.

Once again, we are grateful for the Pearson design team of Tracey Cataldo and Warren Fischbach for their suggestions and expertise.

Our gratitude also goes to Pietro Alongi, Portfolio Director, and Paula Van Els, Content Development Director at Pearson. They were with the series for many years, and we appreciate the support they brought to each new edition.

Our thanks also to our illustrators Chris Pavely and Don Martinetti for their engaging artwork.

Finally, we are grateful for the support of our families as they continue to cheer us on.

Betty S. Azar
Stacy A. Hagen

# Getting Started

 **EXERCISE 1** ▸ **Listening and reading.**
**Part I.** Listen to the conversation between Daniel and Sofia.
They are at a college orientation. They are interviewing each other.

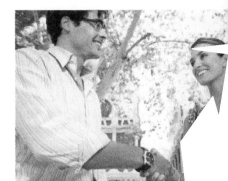

It's Nice to Meet You

DANIEL: Hi. My name is Daniel.

SOFIA: Hi. I'm Sofia. It's nice to meet you.

DANIEL: Nice to meet you too. Where are you from?

SOFIA: I'm from Montreal. How about you?

DANIEL: I'm from Miami.

SOFIA: Are you a new student?

DANIEL: Yes and no. This is my third year of college, but I'm new here.

SOFIA: This is my second year here. I'm in the business school. I really like it.

DANIEL: Oh, my major is economics! Maybe we'll have a class together. So, tell me a little more about yourself. What do you like to do in your free time?

SOFIA: I love the outdoors. I spend a lot of time in the mountains. I hike on weekends. I write about it on social media.

DANIEL: I spend a lot of time outdoors too. I like the beach. In the summer, I swim every day.

SOFIA: This town has a great beach.

DANIEL: Yeah, I want to go there! Now, when I introduce you to the group, I have to write your full name on the board. What's your last name, and how do you spell it?

SOFIA: It's Sanchez. S-A-N-C-H-E-Z.

DANIEL: My last name is Willson — with two "l"s: W-I-L-L-S-O-N.

SOFIA: Oh, it looks like our time is up. I enjoyed our conversation.

DANIEL: Thanks. I enjoyed it too.

**Part II.** Use the information in the conversation to complete Daniel's introduction of Sofia to the class.

DANIEL: I would like to introduce Sofia Sanchez. Sofia is from Montreal. This is her second year of college. In her free time, she...

_____

_____

_____

_____

**Part III.** Now it is Sofia's turn to introduce Daniel. Write her introduction. Begin with *I would like to introduce Daniel Willson*.

_____

_____

_____

_____

## EXERCISE 2 ▶ Let's talk: interview.

**Part I.** Interview a partner.

*Find out your partner's:*

name (and spelling of name)
native country or hometown
free-time activities or hobbies
reason for being here

**Part II.** Introduce your partner to the class. After you learn each student's name, write it down.

## EXERCISE 3 ▶ Writing.

Write answers to the questions. Then, with your teacher, decide what to do with your writing. See the list of suggestions at the end of the exercise.

1. What is your name?
2. Where are you from?
3. Where are you living?
4. Why are you here (in this city)?
   a. Are you a student? If so, what are you studying?
   b. Do you work? If yes, what is your job?
   c. Do you have another reason for being here?
5. What do you like to do in your free time?
6. What is your favorite season of the year? Why?
7. What are your three favorite TV programs or movies? Why do you like them?
8. Describe your first day in this class.

*Suggestions for your writing:*

a. Give it to a classmate to read. Your classmate can then summarize the information in a spoken report to a small group.
b. Work with a partner and correct errors in each other's writing.
c. Read your composition aloud in a small group and answer any questions about it.
d. Hand it in to your teacher, who will correct the errors and return it to you.
e. Hand it in to your teacher, who will return it at the end of the term when your English has gotten better, so you can correct your own errors.

# Connecting Ideas: Punctuation and Meaning

**PRETEST: What do I already know?**
Write "C" if the punctuation, meaning, or verb form is correct. Write "I" if it is incorrect.

1. _____ My mom puts milk lemon and sugar in her tea. (Chart 8-1)

2. _____ Do you prefer coffee or tea with breakfast? (Chart 8-2)

3. _____ Martha had no vacation time, so she was very unhappy. (8-3)

4. _____ Tomorrow won't work for an appointment, but the next day will. (8-4)

5. _____ Joe went to college, but his brother didn't. (8-4)

6. _____ The supervisor doesn't leave work early, and neither don't his employees. (Chart 8-5)

7. _____ Lauren overslept because her alarm didn't ring. (Chart 8-6)

8. _____ Even though Thomas likes to cook, he often eats dinner at home. (Chart 8-7)

9. _____ Jennifer gets good grades although she studies a lot. (Chart 8-7)

**EXERCISE 1 ▶ Warm-up.** (Chart 8-1)
Check (✓) the sentences that have the correct punctuation.

1. _____ I ate some raspberries, and blackberries.

2. _____ I ate some raspberries and blackberries.

3. _____ I ate some raspberries, blackberries, and blueberries.

4. _____ I ate some blueberries, Julia ate some strawberries.

5. _____ I ate some blueberries, and Julia ate some strawberries.

## 8-1 Connecting Ideas with *And*

### Connecting Items within a Sentence

| | |
|---|---|
| (a) NO COMMA: I saw a cat *and* a mouse. <br><br> (b) COMMAS: I saw a cat, a mouse, *and* a dog. | When *and* connects only TWO WORDS (or phrases) within a sentence, NO COMMA is used, as in (a). <br><br> When *and* connects THREE OR MORE items within a sentence, COMMAS are used, as in (b).* |

### Connecting Two Sentences

| | |
|---|---|
| (c) COMMA: I saw a cat, *and* you saw a mouse. | When *and* connects TWO COMPLETE SENTENCES (also called "independent" clauses), a COMMA is usually used, as in (c). |
| (d) PERIOD: I saw a cat. You saw a mouse. <br><br> (e) INCORRECT: *I saw a cat, you saw a mouse.* | Without *and*, two complete sentences are separated by a period, as in (d), *not* a comma.** <br><br> A complete sentence begins with a capital letter; note that *You* is capitalized in (d). |

*In a series of three or more items, the comma before ***and*** is optional. ALSO CORRECT: *I saw a cat, a mouse and a dog.*
**A "period" (the dot used at the end of a sentence) is called a "full stop" in British English.

## EXERCISE 2 ▸ Looking at grammar. (Chart 8-1)

Underline and label the words (noun, verb, adjective) connected by ***and***. Add commas as necessary.

**Birthdays**

1. a. The children gave <u>flowers</u> and <u>gift cards</u> to their grandma. → (*no commas needed*)
     *noun + noun*

   b. The children gave <u>flowers</u>, <u>gift cards</u>, and <u>balloons</u> to their grandma. → (*commas needed*)
     *noun + noun + noun*

2. a. The cake was moist and delicious.

   b. The cake was moist sweet and delicious.

3. a. The girls at the party danced talked and laughed.

   b. The girls at the party danced and talked.

4. a. A clown made dogs cats horses and giraffes out of balloons for the children.

   b. The clown was funny friendly and kind.

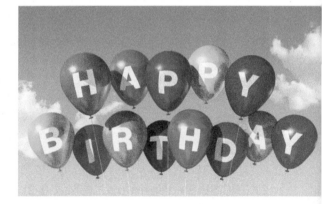

## EXERCISE 3 ▸ Speaking and writing. (Chart 8-1)

Interview another student in your class. Take notes and then write complete sentences using ***and***. Share some of the answers with the class.

*What are ...*

1. your three favorite sports?
2. three adjectives that describe the weather today?
3. four cities that you would like to visit?

4. two characteristics that describe this city or town?

5. five things you did this morning?

6. three things you are afraid of?

7. two or more things that make you happy?

8. the four most important qualities of a good parent?

## EXERCISE 4 ▸ Looking at grammar. (Chart 8-1)
Add commas, periods, and capital letters as necessary.

*Visiting Italy*

1. Italy is a popular country. M̃any tourists go there.

2. Italy is a popular country, and many tourists go there.★

3. High-speed trains run between major cities they are very comfortable.

4. Some interesting cities are Rome Florence Venice Milan and Naples.

5. Milan is in the north Naples is in the south.

6. I asked a question in Italian the tour guide answered in my language.

7. I asked a question in Italian and the tour guide answered in my language.

8. The west coast is beautiful many villages have spectacular views of the sea.

9. You should also visit the east coast Venice is a good place to start.

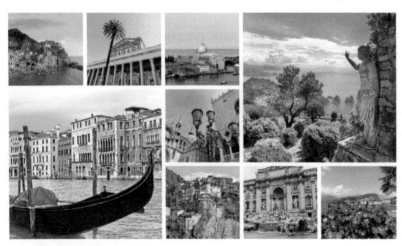

## EXERCISE 5 ▸ Warm-up. (Chart 8-2)
Complete the sentences with your own ideas. Make true statements.

1. When I'm not sure of the meaning of a word in English, I _____ or

   _____.

2. Sometimes I don't understand native speakers of English, but I _____

   _____.

★Sometimes the comma is omitted when **and** connects two very short independent clauses: *The rain fell **and** the wind blew.* In longer sentences, the comma is helpful and usual.

## 8-2 Connecting Ideas with *But* and *Or*

| | |
|---|---|
| (a) I *went* to bed *but couldn't* sleep.<br>(b) Is a lemon *sweet or sour*? | *And*, *but*, and *or* are called "coordinating conjunctions."<br><br>Similar to *and*, *but* and *or* can connect items within a sentence. |
| (c) Did you order *coffee, tea, or milk*?<br>(d) Did you order *coffee, tea or milk*? | When there are three or more items in a series, a comma is used between the first items in the series. A comma before the conjunction is optional, as in (c) and (d). |
| *I dropped the vase.* = a sentence<br>*It didn't break.* = a sentence<br><br>(e) I dropped the vase*, but* it didn't break.<br>(f) Do we have class on Monday*, or* is Monday a holiday? | A comma is usually used when *but* or *or* combines two complete (independent) sentences into one sentence, as in (e) and (f).<br><br>A conjunction can also come at the beginning of a sentence, except in formal writing.<br><br>ALSO CORRECT: I dropped the vase. But it didn't break. I saw a cat. And you saw a mouse. |

### EXERCISE 6 ▸ Looking at grammar. (Charts 8-1 and 8-2)
Complete the sentences with *and, but,* or *or*. Add commas as necessary.

**Sports**

1. Golf __*and*__ tennis are popular sports in my country.
2. Sara is a good tennis player, __*but*__ she doesn't enjoy it.
3. Which would you prefer? Would you like to play tennis __*or*__ golf Saturday?
4. Who won? Did your team _____ the other team score the extra point?
5. Jason doesn't do any exercise _____ he is out of shape. He doesn't care.
6. I got a baseball a basketball _____ a soccer ball for my birthday.
7. Do you like baseball _____ basketball better?
8. I hit the baseball hard _____ it didn't go very far.
9. I play baseball _____ I don't play basketball.
10. Julia kicked the ball _____ didn't score a goal.

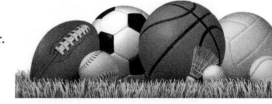

### EXERCISE 7 ▸ Looking at grammar. (Charts 8-1 and 8-2)
Add commas, periods, and capital letters as necessary.

**Electronic Devices\* on Airplanes**

1. Laptops are electronic devices. ᶜcell phones are electronic devices.
2. Laptops and portable DVD players are electronic devices but flashlights aren't.

\**device* = a thing, often electric or electronic, that has a specific purpose

3. In the past, passengers couldn't use these electronic devices during takeoffs and landings they could use them the rest of the flight.

4. Now passengers can use DVD players electronic readers and cell phones for the entire flight but they need to be in airplane mode.

5. Passengers need to put their laptops away for takeoffs and landings they are too big for passengers to hold safely during this time.

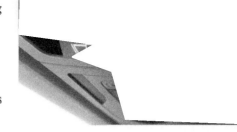

## EXERCISE 8 ▶ Warm-up. (Chart 8-3)
Choose the logical completion for each sentence.

1. I was tired, so I _____.        a. didn't sleep
2. I was tired, but I _____.        b. slept

| 8-3 Connecting Ideas with *So* | |
|---|---|
| (a)  The room was dark, *so* I turned on a light. | **So** can be used as a conjunction, as in (a).  It is preceded by a comma.  It connects the ideas in two independent clauses. <br><br> **So** expresses *results:* <br> cause: *The room was dark.* <br> result: *I turned on a light.* |
| (b)  COMPARE: <br>  The room was dark, *but* I didn't turn on a light. | **But** often expresses an unexpected result, as in (b). |

## EXERCISE 9 ▶ Looking at grammar. (Charts 8-2 and 8-3)
Complete the sentences with *so* or *but*.

**Traffic Problems**

1. a. It began to rain hard, ___*so*___ traffic slowed down.

   b. It began to rain hard, ___*but*___ traffic didn't slow down.

   c. Traffic didn't slow down, _____ there were several accidents.

   d. Traffic didn't slow down, _____ there weren't any accidents.

2. a. The roads were icy, _____ many people drove on them.

   b. The roads were icy, _____ many people took the subway.

3. a. A train hit a car, _____ no one was hurt.

   b. A train hit a car, _____ police closed the road.

   c. Police closed the road, _____ traffic backed up.

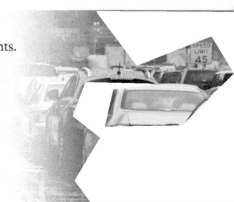

**EXERCISE 10 ▶ Looking at grammar.** (Charts 8-1 → 8-3)
Add commas, periods, and capital letters as necessary.

 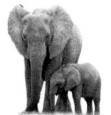

**Surprising Animal Facts**

1. Some tarantulas can go two and a half years without food. <sup>W</sup> when they
   eat, they like grasshoppers beetles small spiders and sometimes small lizards.

2. A female elephant is pregnant for approximately twenty months and almost always has
   only one baby a young elephant stays close to its mother for the first ten years of its life.

3. Dolphins sleep with one eye open they need to be conscious or awake in order to breathe if they
   fall asleep when they are breathing, they will drown so they sleep with half their brain awake and
   one eye open.

 **EXERCISE 11 ▶ Grammar and listening.** (Charts 8-1 → 8-3)
Listen to the passage. Then add commas, periods, and capital letters
as necessary. Listen again as you check your answers.

Do you know these words?
- blinker
- do a good deed
- motioned
- wave someone on

## PAYING IT FORWARD*

(1) <sup>A</sup> a few days ago, a friend and I
were driving from Benton Harbor to
Chicago. <sup>W</sup> we didn't have any delays
for the first hour but we ran into some
highway construction near Chicago
the traffic wasn't moving my friend and
I sat and waited we talked about our
jobs our families and the terrible traffic
slowly it started to move

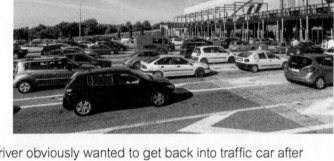

(2) we noticed a black sports car
on the shoulder its blinker was on the driver obviously wanted to get back into traffic car after
car passed without letting him in I decided to do a good deed so I motioned for him to get in line
ahead of me he waved thanks and I waved back at him

(3) all the cars had to stop at a toll booth a short way down the road I held out my money to pay
my toll but the toll-taker just smiled and waved me on she told me that the man in the black sports
car had already paid my toll wasn't that a nice way of saying thank you?

---

*paying it forward = doing something nice for someone after someone does something nice for you. For example, imagine you
are at a coffee stand waiting to buy a cup of coffee. The person in front of you is chatting with you and pays for your cup of
coffee. You then buy a cup of coffee for the next person in line. You are *paying it forward*.

*Paying it forward* means the opposite of *paying it back* (repaying a debt or an obligation).

## EXERCISE 12 ▸ Warm-up. (Chart 8-4)

Complete the sentences. Make true statements. Share a few of your sentences with the class.

1. I like ___fish___, but ___my sister___ doesn't.

2. I don't like _____, but _____ does.

3. I've seen _____, but _____ hasn't.

4. I'm not _____, but _____ is.

5. I wasn't _____ at 1:00 this morning, but _____ was.

6. I will _____, but _____ won't.

---

## 8-4 Using Auxiliary Verbs After *But*

| | |
|---|---|
| (a) I *don't like* coffee, but my husband *does*. | After **but**, often only an auxiliary verb is used. It has the same tense or modal as the main verb. |
| (b) I *like tea*, but my husband *doesn't*. | In (a): **does** = *likes coffee* |
| (c) I *won't be* here tomorrow, but Sue *will*. | |
| (d) I *'ve seen* that movie, but Joe *hasn't*. | Note in the examples: |
| (e) He *isn't here*, but she *is*.* | negative + **but** + affirmative<br>affirmative + **but** + negative |

*A verb is not contracted with a pronoun at the end of a sentence after **but** and **and:**
  CORRECT: ... *but she is.*
  INCORRECT: ... *but she's.*

---

## EXERCISE 13 ▸ Looking at grammar. (Chart 8-4)

**Part I.** Complete each sentence with the correct negative auxiliary verb.

1. Alan listens to podcasts, but his brother ___doesn't___.

2. Alan listens to podcasts, but his brothers ___don't___.

3. Alan is listening to a podcast, but his brother _____.

4. Alan is listening to a podcast, but his brothers _____.

5. Alan listened to a podcast last week, but his brother(s) _____.

6. Alan has listened to some podcasts recently, but his brother _____.

7. Alan has listened to some podcasts recently, but his brothers _____.

8. Alan is going to listen to a podcast soon, but his brother _____.

9. Alan is going to listen to a podcast soon, but his brothers _____.

10. Alan will listen to a podcast soon, but his brother(s) _____.

**Part II.** Complete each sentence with the correct affirmative auxiliary verb.

1. Nicole doesn't use a laptop for her homework, but her sister ___does___.

2. Nicole doesn't use a laptop for her homework, but her sisters ___do___.

3. Nicole isn't using a laptop for her homework, but her sister _____.

4. Nicole isn't using a laptop for her homework, but her sisters _____.

5. Nicole didn't use a laptop for her homework, but her sister(s) _____.

6. Nicole hasn't used a laptop recently, but her sister _____.

7. Nicole hasn't used a laptop recently, but her sisters _____.

8. Nicole isn't going to use a laptop tomorrow, but her sister _____.

9. Nicole isn't going to use a laptop tomorrow, but her sisters _____.

10. Nicole won't use a laptop tomorrow, but her sister(s) _____.

## EXERCISE 14 ▸ Grammar and speaking. (Chart 8-4)

Complete the sentences with true statements about your classmates. You may need to check with them to get more information. Use appropriate auxiliary verbs.

1. ____Kira____ has long hair, but ____Yuki doesn't_____.

2. _____ isn't hungry right now, but _____.

3. _____ lives nearby, but _____.

4. _____ can speak (*a language*) _____ , but _____.

5. _____ plays a musical instrument, but _____.

6. _____ wasn't here last year, but _____.

7. _____ will be at home tonight, but _____.

8. _____ doesn't wear a ring, but _____.

9. _____ didn't study here last year, but _____.

10. _____ has lived here for a long time, but _____.

## EXERCISE 15 ▸ Listening. (Chart 8-4)

Complete the sentences with appropriate auxiliary verbs.

**A Strong Storm**

*Example:* You will hear:  My husband saw a tree fall, but I ...

You will write: ____didn't____ .

1. _____ .          5. _____ .

2. _____ .          6. _____ .

3. _____ .          7. _____ .

4. _____ .          8. _____ .

## EXERCISE 16 ▸ Warm-up. (Chart 8-5)

Match each sentence with the correct picture. NOTE: One picture doesn't match any of the sentences.

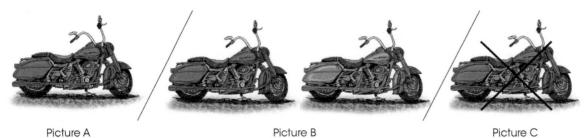

Picture A                    Picture B                    Picture C

1. _____ Alice has a motorcycle, and her husband does too.

2. _____ Alice has a motorcycle, and so does her husband.

3. _____ Alice doesn't have a motorcycle, and her husband doesn't either.

4. _____ Alice doesn't have a motorcycle, and neither does her husband.

| 8-5 | Using *And + Too, So, Either, Neither* |
|---|---|
|                S + AUX + *TOO*<br>(a) Sue works, *and Tom does too*.<br><br>            *SO* + AUX + S<br>(b) Sue works, *and so does Tom*. | In affirmative statements, an auxiliary verb + **too** or **so** can be used after **and**.<br><br>Examples (a) and (b) have the same meaning.<br><br>Word order:<br>   *subject + auxiliary +* **too**<br>   **so**    *+ auxiliary + subject* |
|              S + AUX + *EITHER*<br>(c) Ann doesn't work, *and Joe doesn't either*.<br><br>       *NEITHER* + AUX + S<br>(d) Ann doesn't work, *and neither does Joe*. | An auxiliary verb + **either** or **neither** are used with negative statements.<br><br>Examples (c) and (d) have the same meaning.<br><br>Word order:<br>   *subject + auxiliary +* **either**<br>   **neither** *+ auxiliary + subject*<br><br>NOTE: An affirmative auxiliary is used with *neither*. |
| (e) — I'm hungry.<br>     — *I am too. / So am I.*<br><br>(f) — I never eat meat.<br>     — *I don't either. / Neither do I.* | **And** is not usually used when there are two speakers. |
| (g) — I'm hungry.<br>     — *Me too. (informal)*<br><br>(h) — I never eat meat.<br>     — *Me (n)either. (informal)* | **Me too, me either**, and **me neither** are often used in informal spoken English. |

## EXERCISE 17 ▸ Looking at grammar. (Chart 8-5)

Complete the sentences with the given words. Pay special attention to word order.

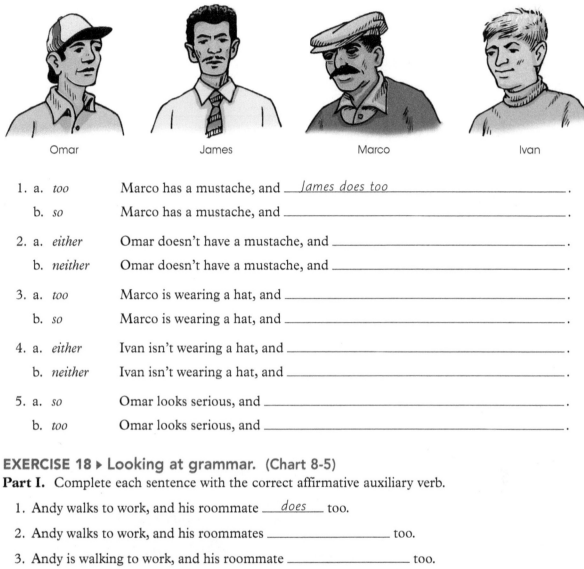

Omar          James          Marco          Ivan

1. a. *too*     Marco has a mustache, and ___*James does too*___.

   b. *so*      Marco has a mustache, and _____.

2. a. *either*  Omar doesn't have a mustache, and _____.

   b. *neither* Omar doesn't have a mustache, and _____.

3. a. *too*     Marco is wearing a hat, and _____.

   b. *so*      Marco is wearing a hat, and _____.

4. a. *either*  Ivan isn't wearing a hat, and _____.

   b. *neither* Ivan isn't wearing a hat, and _____.

5. a. *so*      Omar looks serious, and _____.

   b. *too*     Omar looks serious, and _____.

## EXERCISE 18 ▸ Looking at grammar. (Chart 8-5)

**Part I.** Complete each sentence with the correct affirmative auxiliary verb.

1. Andy walks to work, and his roommate ___*does*___ too.

2. Andy walks to work, and his roommates _____ too.

3. Andy is walking to work, and his roommate _____ too.

4. Andy is walking to work, and his roommates _____ too.

5. Andy walked to work last week, and his roommate(s) _____ too.

6. Andy has walked to work recently, and so _____ his roommate.

7. Andy has walked to work recently, and so _____ his roommates.

8. Andy is going to walk to work tomorrow, and so _____ his roommate.

9. Andy is going to walk to work tomorrow, and so _____ his roommates.

10. Andy will walk to work tomorrow, and so _____ his roommate(s).

**Part II.** Complete each sentence with the correct negative auxiliary verb.

1. Karen doesn't watch TV, and her sister _____*doesn't*_____ either.

2. Karen doesn't watch TV, and her sisters _____ either.

3. Karen isn't watching TV, and her sister _____ either.

4. Karen isn't watching TV, and her sisters _____ either.

5. Karen didn't watch TV last night, and her sister(s) _____ either.

6. Karen hasn't watched TV recently, and neither _____ her sister.

7. Karen hasn't watched TV recently, and neither _____ her sisters.

8. Karen isn't going to watch TV tomorrow, and neither _____ her sister.

9. Karen isn't going to watch TV tomorrow, and neither _____ her sisters.

10. Karen won't watch TV tomorrow, and neither _____ her sister(s).

**EXERCISE 19 ▸ Grammar and speaking. (Chart 8-5)**
Work in small groups. Complete the sentences with ***too, so, either,*** or ***neither***. Make true statements. Answers will vary. You can research information on the internet.

Around the World

1. Haiti is a small country, and _Cuba is too_____.

2. Japan produces rice, and _____.

3. Turkey has had many strong earthquakes, and _____.

4. Iceland doesn't grow coffee, and _____.

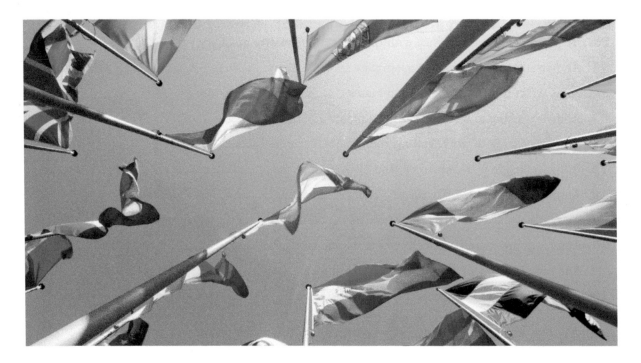

5. Most Canadian children will learn more than one language, and _____.

6. Norway joined the United Nations in 1945, and _____.

7. Argentina doesn't lie on the equator, and _____.

8. Somalia lies on the Indian Ocean, and _____.

9. Monaco has never* hosted the Olympic Games, and _____.

10. South Korea had a Nobel Prize winner in 2000, and _____.

**EXERCISE 20 ▶ Let's talk: pairwork.** (Chart 8-5)
Work with a partner. Partner A says a sentence. Partner B agrees with Speaker A's statement by using **so** or **neither**. Take turns.

*Example:* I'm confused.
PARTNER A (*book open*):   I'm confused.
PARTNER B (*book closed*):   So am I.

| PARTNER A | PARTNER B |
|---|---|
| 1. I studied last night. | 1. I overslept this morning. |
| 2. I study grammar every day. | 2. I don't like mushrooms. |
| 3. I'd like a cup of coffee. | 3. Swimming is an Olympic sport. |
| 4. I'm not hungry. | 4. Denmark doesn't have any volcanoes. |
| 5. I've never seen a vampire. | 5. I've never seen a ghost. |
| 6. Running is an aerobic activity. | 6. Chickens lay eggs. |
| 7. Snakes don't have legs. | 7. Elephants can swim. |
| 8. Coffee contains caffeine. | 8. I'd rather go to (*name of a place*) than (*name of a place*). |

**EXERCISE 21 ▶ Listening and speaking.** (Chart 8-5)
**Part I.** There are responses you can use if you want to get more information or if you disagree with someone else's statement. Listen to the examples. Pay special attention to the sentence stress in items 4–6 when Speaker B is disagreeing.

*To get more information:*
1. A: I'm going to drop this class.
   B: **You are?  Why?  What's the matter?**

2. A: My phone doesn't have enough memory for this app.
   B: **Really?  Are you sure?**

3. A: I can read Braille.
   B: **You can?  How did you learn to do that?**

*To disagree:*
4. A: I love this weather.
   B: **I don't.**

---

*Never makes a sentence negative: *The teacher is **never** late, and **neither** am I.* OR *I'm **not either.**

5. A: I didn't like the movie.

   B: **I did!**

6. A: I'm excited about graduation.

   B: **I'm not.**

**Part II.** Work with a partner. Partner A will make a statement, and Partner B will ask for more information. Take turns saying the sentences.

1. I'm feeling tired.
2. I don't like grammar.
3. I've seen a ghost.
4. I didn't eat breakfast this morning.
5. I haven't slept well all week.
6. I'm going to leave class early.

**Part III.** Now take turns disagreeing with the statements.

7. I believe in ghosts.
8. I didn't study hard for the last test.
9. I'm going to exercise for an hour today.
10. I like strawberries.
11. I haven't worked very hard this week.
12. I don't enjoy birthdays.

## EXERCISE 22 ▶ Grammar and speaking. (Charts 8-4 and 8-5)

Make true statements about your classmates using *and* and *but*. You may need to interview them to get more information. Use the appropriate auxiliary verbs. Share some of your sentences with the class.

1. _____*Kunio*_____ lives in an apartment, and _____*Boris does too*_____ .

2. _____*Ellen*_____ is wearing jeans, but _____*Ricardo isn't*_____ .

3. _____ is absent today, but _____ .

4. _____ didn't teach English last year, and _____ either.

5. _____ can cook, and _____ too.

6. _____ has a baseball cap, and _____ too.

7. _____ doesn't have a motorcycle, and _____ either.

8. _____ doesn't have a pet, but _____ .

9. _____ will get up early tomorrow, but _____ .

10. _____ has studied English for more than a year, and _____ too.

**EXERCISE 23** ▸ Warm-up.  (Chart 8-6)
Choose all the logical completions.

Because Roger felt tired, _____ .

    a. he took a nap.
    b. he didn't take a nap.
    c. he went to bed early.
    d. he didn't go to bed early.

## 8-6 Connecting Ideas with *Because*

| | | |
|---|---|---|
| (a) | He drank water *because* he was thirsty. | ***Because*** expresses a cause; it gives a reason.  Why did he drink water? *Reason:*  He was thirsty. |
| (b) | MAIN CLAUSE: *He drank water.* | A main clause is a complete sentence:  ***He drank water*** = a complete sentence |
| (c) | ADVERB CLAUSE: *because he was thirsty* | An adverb clause is NOT a complete sentence:  ***because he was thirsty*** = NOT a complete sentence  ***Because*** introduces an adverb clause:  ***because*** + *subject* + *verb* = *an adverb clause* |
| (d) | MAIN CLAUSE   ADVERB CLAUSE<br>He drank water *because he was thirsty*.<br>(no comma)<br><br>ADVERB CLAUSE   MAIN CLAUSE<br>(e) *Because he was thirsty,* he drank water.<br>(comma) | An adverb clause is connected to a main clause, as in (d) and (e).<br>In (d): *main clause + no comma + adverb clause*<br>In (e): *adverb clause + comma + main clause*<br>Examples (d) and (e) have exactly the same meaning. |
| (f) | INCORRECT IN WRITING:<br>He drank water. *Because he was thirsty.* | Example (f) is incorrect in written English: ***Because he was thirsty*** cannot stand alone as a sentence that starts with a capital letter and ends with a period.  It has to be connected to a main clause, as in (d) and (e). |
| (g) | CORRECT IN SPEAKING:<br>— Why did he drink some water?<br>— Because he was thirsty. | In spoken English, an adverb clause can be used as the short answer to a question, as in (g). |

**EXERCISE 24** ▸ Looking at grammar.  (Chart 8-6)
Combine each pair of sentences in two different orders.  Use ***because***.  Punctuate carefully.

**Tom's car is a lemon!**

1. Tom knew he bought a lemon. \ He had problems the first week.
   → *Tom knew he bought a lemon because he had problems the first week.*
   → *Because he had problems the first week, Tom knew he bought a lemon.*

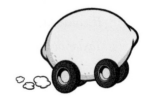

2. The battery was dead. \ His car didn't start the other day.

3. The Check Engine light is on. \ The car is leaking oil.

4. The heater isn't working. \ It's freezing inside.

5. The windows are foggy. \ The defroster is broken.

**EXERCISE 25 ▸ Looking at grammar.** (Chart 8-6)
Add periods, commas, and capital letters as necessary.

Nighttime Fears

1. Jimmy is very young. *B*because he is afraid of the dark, he likes to have a light on in his bedroom at night.

2. Andrew thinks a wolf lives under his bed because he is so scared his dad looks under his bed every night.

3. Kim believes a ghost lives in her bedroom closet because she thinks the ghost comes out at night she sleeps with the closet door closed.

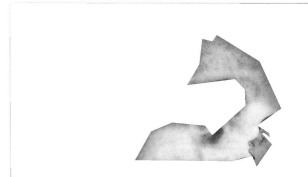

4. Lesley is afraid of spiders in her bed because she once saw a spider web over her bed she checks under her covers every night.

**EXERCISE 26 ▸ Looking at grammar.** (Charts 8-3 and 8-6)
**Part I.** Restate the sentences, paying attention to punctuation. Use *so*.

Making Decisions

1. Alberto is meeting with his advisor because he hasn't decided on a major.

   → *Alberto hasn't decided on a major, so he is meeting with his advisor.*

2. Because Clarita has trouble making decisions, she calls her mom every day for advice.

3. Julia is a popular manager because she asks her employees for their opinions before she makes important decisions.

**Part II.** Restate the sentences, paying attention to punctuation. Use ***because***.

4. Taylor's parents were very controlling, so she doesn't have much experience making decisions.

   → *Because Taylor's parents were very controlling, she doesn't have much experience making decisions.*

   → *Taylor doesn't have much experience making decisions because her parents were very controlling.*

5. Annika likes to think about the pros and cons of a problem, so she doesn't make decisions quickly.

6. Jonathan thinks he knows everything, so he never asks anyone for advice.

### EXERCISE 27 ▸ Looking at grammar. (Charts 8-1 → 8-6)

Add commas, periods, and capital letters as necessary. Don't change any of the words or the order of the words.

Cooling Off

1. Jim was hot. *H*̷e sat in the shade.

2. Jim was hot and tired so he sat in the shade.

3. Jim was hot tired and thirsty.

4. Because he was hot Jim sat in the shade.

5. Because they were hot and thirsty Jim and Susan sat in the shade and drank iced-tea.

6. Jim and Susan sat in the shade and drank iced-tea because they were hot and thirsty.

7. Jim sat in the shade drank iced-tea and fanned himself with his cap because he was hot tired and thirsty.

8. Because Jim was hot he stayed under the shade of the tree but Susan went back to work.

### EXERCISE 28 ▸ Grammar and listening. (Charts 8-1 → 8-6)

Add commas, periods, and capital letters as necessary.
Then listen to the passage to help you check your answers.

Do you know these words?
- allergies      - sneeze
- dust           - metal
- flower pollen  - itch
                 - reaction

# STRANGE ALLERGIES

Allergies make people sneeze, cough, itch, or turn red. *C*ommon causes of allergies are dust flower pollen animal fur and nuts there are other things that cause allergies but they are not so well known dark chocolate can make some people sneeze the metal in cell phones can cause some people's skin to turn red and itch cold weather and leather clothing can also cause redness and itching in some people.

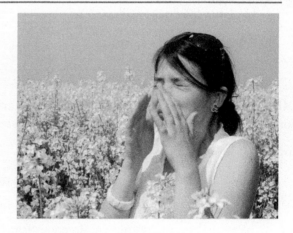

## EXERCISE 29 ▸ Warm-up. (Chart 8-7)

In which sentences is the result (in green) the opposite of what you expect?

1. Even though Silvia took a cooking class, she often burns the food.
2. Because Silvia burned the food, no one wanted to eat it.
3. Although Silvia took a cooking class, she often burns the food.

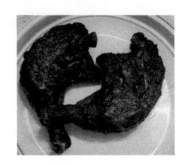

| 8-7 | Connecting Ideas with *Even Though/Although* | |
|---|---|---|
| (a) | *Even though* I was hungry, I did not eat. <br> I did not eat *even though* I was hungry. | ***Even though*** and ***although*** introduce an adverb clause. |
| (b) | *Although* I was hungry, I did not eat. <br> I did not eat *although* I was hungry. | Examples (a) and (b) have the same meaning: <br> *I was hungry, but I did not eat.* |
| COMPARE: | | |
| (c) | *Because*　　I was hungry, *I ate.* | ***Because*** expresses an expected result, as in (c). |
| (d) | *Even though*　　I was hungry, *I did not eat.* | ***Even though/although*** expresses an unexpected or opposite result, as in (d). |

## EXERCISE 30 ▸ Looking at grammar. (Chart 8-7)

Complete the sentences with the words in *italics*.

1. *is / isn't*

    a. Because Dan is sick, he ＿＿＿＿＿＿ going to work.

    b. Although Dan is sick, he ＿＿＿＿＿＿ going to work.

    c. Even though Dan is sick, he ＿＿＿＿＿＿ going to work.

2. *went / didn't go*

    a. Even though it was late, we ＿＿＿＿＿＿＿ home.

    b. Although it was late, we ＿＿＿＿＿＿＿ home.

    c. Because it was late, we ＿＿＿＿＿＿＿ home.

## EXERCISE 31 ▸ Looking at grammar. (Chart 8-7)

Complete the sentences with **even though** or **because**.

Special Talents

1. *Because*＿＿＿＿ Po has a photographic memory, he does well on tests.

2. *Even though*＿＿＿ Po has a photographic memory, his grades aren't good.

3. ＿＿＿＿＿＿＿ Amir can do complicated math in his head, he doesn't understand geometry.

4. ＿＿＿＿＿＿＿ Janette can draw a perfect circle, her teacher asks her to draw shapes on the board.

5. _____ Sabrina can do magic tricks, people ask her to entertain at parties.

6. _____ Alberto can crack an egg with one hand, he uses two.

7. _____ Philip can't read music, he can play the piano perfectly.

8. _____ Lilly can juggle several objects at one time, she is popular with children.

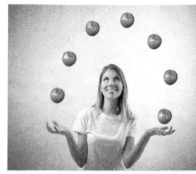

## EXERCISE 32 ▸ Looking at grammar. (Charts 8-6 and 8-7)

Choose the best completion for each sentence.

1. Even though the test was fairly easy, most of the class _____.
   a. failed
   b. passed
   c. did pretty well

2. Jack hadn't heard or read about the bank robbery even though _____.
   a. he was the robber
   b. it was all over social media
   c. he was out of town when it occurred

3. Although _____, she finished the race in first place.
   a. Miki was full of energy and strength
   b. Miki was leading all the way
   c. Miki was far behind in the beginning

4. We can see the light from an airplane at night before we can hear the plane because _____.
   a. light travels faster than sound
   b. airplanes travel at high speeds
   c. our eyes work better than our ears at night

5. My partner and I worked all day and late into the evening. Even though _____, we stopped at our favorite restaurant before we went home.
   a. we were very hungry
   b. we had finished our report
   c. we were very tired

6. Although Jenna says she is vegetarian, she _____.
   a. eats meat
   b. doesn't eat meat
   c. eats a lot of vegetables

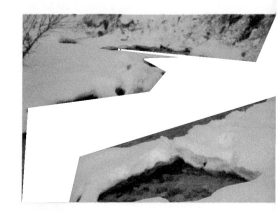

7. In the spring, the snow melts into mountain rivers. The water carries dirt and rocks. Mountain rivers turn brown because _____.
   a. mountains have a lot of snow
   b. the water from melting snow brings soil and rocks to the river
   c. ice is frozen water

**EXERCISE 33 ▸ Listening.** (Charts 8-6 and 8-7)
Choose the best completion for each sentence.

*Example:* You will hear:   Because there was a sale at the mall, …
        You will choose:   a. it wasn't busy.
                        (b.) there were a lot of shoppers.
                        c. prices were very high.

1. a. they were under some mail.
  b. my roommate helped me look for them.
  c. I never found them.

2. a. the rain had stopped.
  b. a storm was coming.
  c. the weather was nice.

3. a. he was feeling sick.
  b. he wanted to.
  c. he was happy for me.

4. a. I mailed it.
  b. I decided not to mail it.
  c. I sent it to a friend.

5. a. Carlo bought a big car.
  b. Carlo doesn't take the bus.
  c. Carlo drives a small car.

6. a. the coaches celebrated afterwards.
  b. the fans cheered loudly.
  c. the players didn't seem very excited.

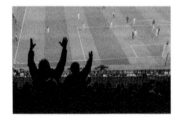

**EXERCISE 34 ▸ Let's talk.** (Charts 8-6 and 8-7)
Answer the questions in complete sentences. Use either **because** or **even though**. Work in pairs, in small groups, or as a class.

*Example:* Last night you were tired. Did you go to bed early?
  → *Yes, I went to bed early because I was tired.* OR
  → *Yes, because I was tired, I went to bed before nine.* OR
  → *No, I didn't go to bed early even though I was really tired.* OR
  → *No, even though I was really tired, I didn't go to bed until after midnight.*

1. Last night you were tired. Did you stay up late?
2. Vegetables are good for you. Do you eat a lot of them?
3. Space exploration is exciting. Would you like to be an astronaut?
4. What are the winters like here? Do you like living here in the winter?
5. (*A recent movie*) has had good reviews. Do you want to see it?
6. Are you a good artist? Will you draw a picture of me on the board?
7. Where does your family live? Are you going to visit them over the next holiday?

**EXERCISE 35 ▶ Reading and grammar. (Chapter 8 Review)**
**Part I.** Read the blog entry by co-author Stacy Hagen.

# BlackBookBlog

## Choking Under Pressure

Do tests make you nervous? If they do, you are not alone. Many students become very nervous, and this causes problems during the test. They sometimes can't think, or they forget information that they studied. English has an idiom for this: They "choke under pressure." Usually, we use the word *choke* when we talk about eating. The food doesn't go down our throats, and we can't breathe correctly. "Choking under pressure" means that we do poorly, for example, at school or in sports.

Psychologist Sian Beilock wrote a book called *Choke*. Beilock says that thinking too much, or overthinking, is the problem. Imagine some baseball players. Their team needs to score, and they are thinking about how to do this. They want to hit, throw, or catch the ball really well, and they begin to worry. This takes energy. Our minds don't do two things well, such as playing and worrying, at the same time. When we worry, we may not do the other activity well.

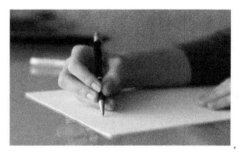

Beilock says the same is true for test-taking. In one of her studies, students took ten minutes to write down their worries before they took a test. They scored higher than students who didn't. Beilock says that by writing thoughts down, students identify their worries. They may see that the situation is not so bad and that they can deal with it. This helps them worry less when they take the test.

Of course, athletes can't stop and write down their thoughts. Beilock recommends that they think about something else. For example, a baseball player can look at the stitching on the ball. That can stop him or her from worrying about throwing a really good ball or winning the game.

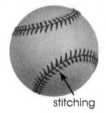
stitching

The next time you feel the pressure of a test or sporting event, try one of Beilock's techniques. There is a good chance you will feel more relaxed when you are able to identify the worry or think about something else.

**Part II.** Complete the sentences with words and phrases in the box. More than one answer may be correct. Add punctuation as necessary.

| | | | |
|---|---|---|---|
| students | want to do well | they forget information | they begin to worry |
| athletes | identify their worries | they choke | they sometimes do poorly |

1. _____ and _____ can choke under pressure.

2. Some students get very nervous before a test so _____.

3. Nervous students _____ but _____ .

4. Because athletes think about doing really well _____ .

5. Students can write their thoughts down and _____ .

6. Even though athletes and students prepare very well _____ .

7. Although people often try to do better by thinking about doing well _____ .

## EXERCISE 36 ▸ Check your knowledge. (Chapter 8 Review)

Correct the errors in sentence structure. Pay special attention to punctuation.

1. Even though I was sick, but I went to work.

2. Gold silver and copper. They are metals.

3. The children crowded around the teacher. Because he was doing a magic trick.

4. I had a cup of coffee, and so does my friend.

5. My roommate didn't go. Neither I went either.

6. Even I was exhausted, I didn't stop working until after midnight.

7. Although I like chocolate, but I can't eat it because I'm allergic to it.

8. I like to eat eggs for breakfast and everybody else in my family too.

9. A home improvement store sells tools and paint and flooring and appliances.

10. Most insects have wings, spiders do not.

## EXERCISE 37 ▸ Writing. (Chapter 8)

**Part I.** Write about an animal that interests you. Follow these steps:

1. Choose an animal you want to know more about.

    *Hint*: If you are doing your research on the internet, type in "interesting facts about _____ " (*name of animal*).

2. Take notes on the information you find. For example, here is some information about giraffes from an internet site.

    *Sample notes:*

    Giraffes …
    → have long necks (6 feet or 1.8 meters)
    → can reach the tops of trees
    → need very little sleep (20 minutes to two hours out of 24 hours)
    → eat about 140 pounds of food a day
    → can go for weeks without drinking water
    → get a lot of water from the plants they eat
    → can grab and hold onto objects with their tongues
    → don't have vocal cords
    → can communicate with one another (but humans can't hear them)

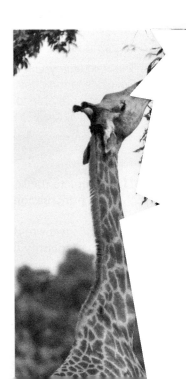

→ are now having a hard time living in the wild. (There are only 80,000 left and the population is getting smaller.)
→ need protection

3. Write sentences based on your facts. Combine some of the ideas using *and, but, or, so, because, although, even though*.

*Sample sentences:*

→ Giraffes have long necks, so they can reach the tops of trees.
→ Although they eat about 140 pounds of food a day, they can go for weeks without drinking water.
→ Even though giraffes don't have vocal cords, they can communicate with one another.
→ Giraffes can communicate, but people can't hear their communication.

4. Put your sentences into a paragraph, with a topic sentence, logical order of ideas, and a concluding sentence.

*Sample paragraph:*

**Interesting Facts About Giraffes**

Giraffes are interesting animals. They have long necks, so they can reach the tops of trees. They eat flowers, fruit, climbing plants, and the twigs and leaves from trees. Although they eat about 140 pounds of food a day, they can go for weeks without drinking water. But they get water from the plants they eat too. They have very long tongues, and these tongues are useful. Because they are so long, they can grab objects with them. Even though giraffes don't have vocal cords, they can communicate. The noises are very low, and people can't hear them. Giraffe populations are getting smaller. There are about 80,000 left in the world, and to survive, these amazing creatures need protection.

---

**WRITING TIP**

In addition to a topic sentence and major (big) details, paragraphs also have minor (small) details. The minor details add more information to the major detail:

**Major:**  They have long necks, so they can reach the tops of trees.
**Minor:**  They eat flowers, fruit, climbing plants, and the twigs and leaves from trees.

**Major:**  They have very long tongues, and these tongues are useful.
**Minor:**  Because they are so long, they can grab objects with them.

Your writing is stronger if you have at least one additional sentence to support each major detail.

---

**Part II.** Edit your writing. Check for the following:

1. ☐ use of connecting words: *and, but, or, so, because, even though, although*
2. ☐ correct punctuation with connecting words
3. ☐ a topic sentence and a concluding sentence
4. ☐ enough minor details to support all major details
5. ☐ correct spelling (use a dictionary or spell-check)

---

▪▪▪▪▪ For digital resources, go to the Pearson Practice English app.

**PRETEST: What do I already know?**
Write "C" if the **boldfaced** words are correct and "I" if they are incorrect.

1. _____ What is **more good** to have: high grades or good test scores? (Chart 9-1)

2. _____ Is love **more importanter than** money? (Chart 9-1)

3. _____ My hometown has **the friendliest people in** my country. (Chart 9-2)

4. _____ Lisa works **harder than** her co-workers do. (Chart 9-3)

5. _____ **One of the longest river in the world** is the Yangtze River in China. (Chart 9-3)

6. _____ Silvia is a fast driver. She **drives more fastly than** her husband. (Chart 9-4)

7. _____ **The longer** Daniel talked, **the more excited** he became. (Chart 9-5)

8. _____ My grandfather is **very healthier** than my grandmother. (Chart 9-6)

9. _____ This dessert has a lot of sugar. I've never tasted **a sweeter** dessert. (Chart 9-7)

10. _____ English is **as hard as** math for me. (Chart 9-8)

11. _____ A compact car is **not as large as** an SUV (sport utility vehicle). (Chart 9-9)

12. _____ There are **more vegetables** in the garden this year **than** last year. (Chart 9-10)

13. _____ You look **the same like** your brother. (Chart 9-11)

**EXERCISE 1 ▶ Warm-up.** (Chart 9-1)
Compare the people.

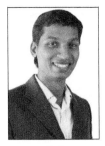
Raj

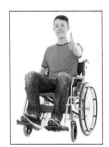
Daniel

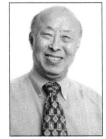
Taka

1. Raj looks younger than _____.

2. Daniel looks younger than _____.

3. Taka looks older than _____.

## 9-1 Introduction to Comparative Forms of Adjectives

| (a) "A" is *older than* "B."<br>(b) "A" and "B" are *older than* "C" and "D."<br>(c) Ed is *more generous than* his brother. | The comparative compares *this* to *that* or *these* to *those*.<br><br>Form: **-er** or **more**<br><br>NOTE: A comparative is followed by **than**. |
|---|---|

|  | ADJECTIVE | COMPARATIVE |  |
|---|---|---|---|
| ONE-SYLLABLE ADJECTIVES | old<br>wise | **older**<br>**wiser** | For most one-syllable adjectives, **-er** is added. |
| TWO-SYLLABLE ADJECTIVES | famous<br>pleasant | **more famous**<br>**more pleasant** | For most two-syllable adjectives, **more** is used. |
|  | clever<br>gentle<br>friendly | **cleverer/more clever**<br>**gentler/more gentle**<br>**friendlier/more friendly** | Some two-syllable adjectives use either **-er** or **more**: *able, angry, clever, common, cruel, friendly, gentle, handsome, narrow, pleasant, polite, quiet, simple, sour.* |
|  | busy<br>pretty | **busier**<br>**prettier** | **-Er** is used with two-syllable adjectives that end in **-y**. The **-y** is changed to **-i**. |
| ADJECTIVES WITH THREE OR MORE SYLLABLES | important<br>fascinating | **more important**<br>**more fascinating** | **More** is used with long adjectives.<br>NOTE: The opposite of **more** is **less**:<br>        *less important, less fascinating* |
| IRREGULAR ADJECTIVES | good<br>bad | **better**<br>**worse** | **Good** and **bad** have irregular comparative forms. |

## EXERCISE 2 ▸ Looking at grammar. (Chart 9-1)

Complete the sentences with comparisons. Think about people, places, school subjects, and objects. Use **is** or **are** for the verbs. Share a few of your answers with the class.

*In my opinion ...*

1. _____ harder than _____ .
2. _____ more beautiful than _____ .
3. _____ more interesting than _____ .
4. _____ more exciting than _____ .
5. _____ safer than _____ .
6. _____ more famous than _____ .
7. _____ more important than _____ .
8. _____ more useful than _____ .
9. _____ simpler than _____ .
10. _____ better than _____ .

## EXERCISE 3 ▸ Looking at grammar. (Chart 9-1)

Write the comparative forms for these adjectives.

1. healthy     _healthier than_ _____
2. difficult     _____
3. easy     _____
4. boring     _____
5. dangerous     _____
6. cold     _____
7. pretty     _____
8. relaxing     _____
9. funny     _____
10. bad     _____
11. angry     _____
12. lazy     _____
13. quiet     _____
14. hot     _____

## EXERCISE 4 ▸ Game: trivia. (Chart 9-1)

Work in teams. Complete each sentence with the correct comparative form of the adjective. Then decide if the sentences are true (T) or false (F). The team with the most correct answers wins.*

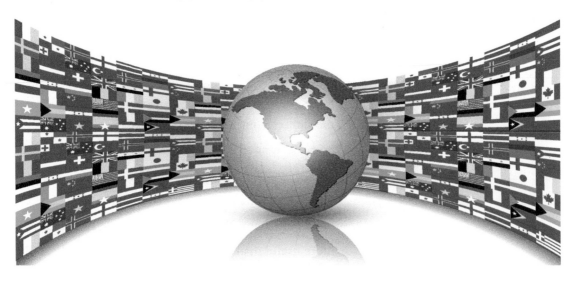

1. Canada is (*large*) _____ than France.     T  F
2. The South Pole is generally (*cold*) _____ than the North Pole.     T  F

---

*See *Trivia Answers*, p. 443.

3. Africa is (*big*) _____ than Asia.  T  F

4. In general, Libya is (*hot*) _____ than Mexico.  T  F

5. London is (*wet*) _____ than Madrid.  T  F

6. The Atlantic Ocean is (*deep*) _____ than the Pacific Ocean.  T  F

7. Malaysia is (*humid*) _____ than Paris.  T  F

8. Canada is (*crowded*) _____ than China.  T  F

9. The Nile River is (*long*) _____ than the Mississippi River.  T  F

10. The Andes Mountains are (*high*) _____ than the
Himalaya Mountains.  T  F

**EXERCISE 5 ▸ Looking at grammar.** (Chart 9-1)
Complete the sentences with the correct comparative form (***more/-er***) of the adjectives
in the box.

| | | | |
|---|---|---|---|
| clean | dangerous | funny | ✓ sweet |
| confusing | dark | pretty | wet |

1. Oranges are _____ *sweeter* _____ than lemons.

2. I heard some polite laughter when I told my jokes, but everyone laughed loudly when Janet told
hers.  Her jokes are always _____ than mine.

3. Many more people die in car accidents than in plane accidents.  Statistics show that driving your
own car is _____ than flying in an airplane.

4. Professor Sato speaks clearly, but I have trouble understanding Professor Larson's lectures.
Professor Larson's lectures are much _____ than Professor Sato's.

5. Is there a storm coming?  The sky looks _____ than it did an hour ago.

6. That tablecloth has some stains on it.  Take this one.  It's _____ .

7. We're having another beautiful sunrise.  It looks like an orange fireball.  The sky is even
_____ than yesterday.

8. If a cat and a duck are out in the rain, the cat
will get much _____ than
the duck.  The water will just roll off the duck's
feathers, but it will soak into the cat's hair.

**EXERCISE 6 ▸ Let's talk: pairwork. (Chart 9-1)**

Work with a partner. Make comparisons with *more*/-*er* and the adjectives in the box. Share some of your answers with the class.

Opinions

| | | | |
|---|---|---|---|
| beautiful | enjoyable | light | soft |
| cheap | expensive | relaxing | stressful |
| deep | fast | shallow | thick |
| easy | heavy | short | thin |

1. traveling by air \ traveling by train
   → *Traveling by air is faster than traveling by train.*
   → *Traveling by air is more stressful than traveling by train.*
      Etc.
2. a pool \ a lake
3. a final exam \ a quiz
4. taking a trip \ staying home
5. iron furniture \ wood furniture
6. going to the doctor \ going to the dentist
7. gold jewelry \ silver jewelry
8. plastic toys \ wood toys
9. an emerald \ a diamond
10. a feather \ a blade of grass

**EXERCISE 7 ▸ Listening. (Chart 9-1)**

Listen to the statements. Do you agree or disagree? Circle *yes* or *no*.

Opinions

| 1. yes | no | 5. yes | no |
|---|---|---|---|
| 2. yes | no | 6. yes | no |
| 3. yes | no | 7. yes | no |
| 4. yes | no | 8. yes | no |

Do you know these words?
- raw
- history

**EXERCISE 8 ▸ Warm-up. (Chart 9-2)**

Compare the three handwriting samples.

A: *The meeting starts at eight!*

B: *The meeting starts at eight :*

C: *The meeting starts at eight!*

1. __C__ is neater than __A (or B)__ .
2. _____ is messier than _____ .
3. _____ is the messiest.
4. _____ is the best.
5. _____ is the worst.

## 9-2 Introduction to Superlative Forms of Adjectives

| | | |
|---|---|---|
| (a) "A," "B," "C," and "D" are sisters. "A" is *the oldest of all* four sisters. | The superlative compares one person or one part of a whole group to all the rest of the group. | |
| (b) A woman in Turkey claims to be *the oldest person in the world*. | Form: *-est* or *most* | |
| (c) Ed is *the most generous person in his family*. | NOTE: A superlative begins with *the*. | |

| | ADJECTIVE | SUPERLATIVE | |
|---|---|---|---|
| ONE-SYLLABLE ADJECTIVES | old<br>wise | **the oldest**<br>**the wisest** | For most one-syllable adjectives, *-est* is added. |
| TWO-SYLLABLE ADJECTIVES | famous<br>pleasant | **the most famous**<br>**the most pleasant** | For most two-syllable adjectives, *most* is used. |
| | clever<br><br>gentle<br><br>friendly | **the cleverest**<br>**the most clever**<br>**the gentlest**<br>**the most gentle**<br>**the friendliest**<br>**the most friendly** | Some two-syllable adjectives use either *-est* or *most*: *able, angry, clever, common, cruel, friendly, gentle, handsome, narrow, pleasant, polite, quiet, simple, sour.* |
| | busy<br>pretty | **the busiest**<br>**the prettiest** | *-Est* is used with two-syllable adjectives that end in *-y*. The *-y* is changed to *-i*. |
| ADJECTIVES WITH THREE OR MORE SYLLABLES | important<br>fascinating | **the most important**<br>**the most fascinating** | *Most* is used with long adjectives.<br>NOTE: The opposite of *most* is *least*:<br>   *the least important, the least fascinating* |
| IRREGULAR ADJECTIVES | good<br>bad | **the best**<br>**the worst** | *Good* and *bad* have irregular superlative forms. |

## EXERCISE 9 ▶ Looking at grammar. (Charts 9-1 and 9-2)

Write the comparative and superlative forms of the following adjectives.

1. high    *higher, the highest*
2. good    _____
3. lazy    _____
4. hot★    _____
5. neat★    _____
6. late★    _____
7. sweet    _____

8. dangerous    _____
9. slow    _____
10. common    _____
11. friendly    _____
12. careful    _____
13. bad    _____
14. ugly    _____

---

★Spelling notes:
- When a one-syllable adjective ends in *one vowel + a consonant*, double the consonant and add *-er/-est: sad, sadder, saddest* (except for adjectives that end in *-e: wide, wider, widest*).
- When an adjective ends in *two vowels + a consonant*, do NOT double the consonant: *cool, cooler, coolest.*

**EXERCISE 10 ▶ Game: trivia. (Chart 9-2)**

Work in teams. Make true sentences with the given words. Use superlatives. The team with the most correct answers wins.*

In the World

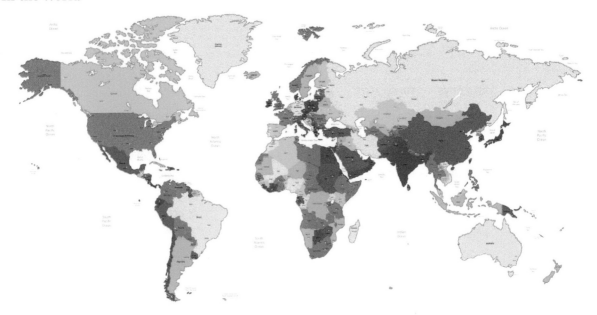

**Oceans:** *the Atlantic / the Pacific / the Arctic / the Indian*

1. (*deep*) _____The deepest ocean is the Pacific.___ OR _The Pacific is the deepest ocean.___

2. (*cold*) _____

3. (*big*) _____

**Continents:** *Africa / Antarctica / Australia / Asia / South America*

4. (*windy*) _____

5. (*hot*) _____

6. (*populated*) _____

**Countries in Asia:** *India / China / Singapore / the Maldives*

7. (*large*) _____

8. (*small*) _____

**Mountains:** *Denali / Mount Fuji / Mount Kilimanjaro / Mount Blanc*

9. (*tall*) _____

10. (*low*) _____

**Animals:** *the whale / the elephant / the greyhound dog / the cheetah / the kangaroo*

11. (*heavy*) _____

12. (*fast*) _____

*See *Trivia Answers*, p. 443.

## EXERCISE 11 ▶ Looking at grammar. (Chart 9-2)

Complete the sentences with your own words and the superlative form of the words in parentheses. Share a few of your answers with the class.

**In My Opinion**

1. (*difficult*) ___Physics___ is ___the most difficult___ subject.
2. (*easy*) _____ is _____ class.
3. (*good*) _____ is _____ time for me to fall asleep.
4. (*bad*) _____ is _____ food I have ever eaten.
5. (*happy*) _____ is _____ person in my family.
6. (*neat*) _____ is _____ person in my family.
7. (*interesting*) _____ is _____ athlete right now.
8. (*busy*) _____ is _____ person I know.

## EXERCISE 12 ▶ Let's talk: interview. (Chart 9-2)

Make questions with the given words and the superlative form. Then interview your classmates, and share some of their answers with the class.

1. what \ bad movie \ you have ever seen

   → *What is the worst movie you have ever seen?*

2. what \ interesting sport to watch \ on TV
3. what \ crowded city \ you have ever visited
4. where \ good restaurant \ around here
5. what \ fun place to visit \ in this area
6. who \ kind person \ you know
7. what \ important thing \ in life
8. what \ serious problem \ in the world
9. who \ interesting person \ in the news right now

## EXERCISE 13 ▶ Listening. (Charts 9-1 and 9-2)

The endings **-er** and **-est** can be hard to hear. Listen to the sentences and choose the words that you hear.

**My Family**

***Example:*** You will hear:     I am the shortest person in our family.

You will choose:   short    shorter   (shortest)

1. short      shorter      shortest
2. tall       taller       tallest
3. happy      happier      happiest
4. happy      happier      happiest
5. old        older        oldest
6. funny      funnier      funniest
7. wise       wiser        wisest
8. wise       wiser        wisest

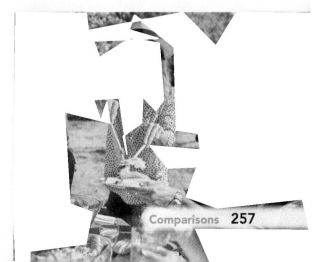

**EXERCISE 14 ▸ Warm up.  (Chart 9-3)**
Complete the sentences with true information.

1. _____ is the oldest person in my family/group of friends.

2. I'm older than _____ is.

3. _____ is one of the oldest people I know.

| 9-3 | Completing Comparatives and Superlatives |
|---|---|
| (a) I'm older *than my brother* (is). <br> (b) I'm older *than he is.* <br> (c) I'm older *than him.*  (*informal*) | In formal English, a subject pronoun (e.g., *he*) follows **than**, as in (b). <br> In informal spoken English, you may sometimes hear an object pronoun (e.g., *him*) after **than**, as in (c). |
| (d) *Ann's* hair is longer *than Kate's.* <br> (e) *Jack's* apartment is smaller *than mine.* | A possessive noun (e.g., *Kate's*) or pronoun (e.g., *mine*) may follow **than**. |
| (f) Tokyo is one of *the largest cities in the world.* <br> (g) David is *the most generous person I have ever known.* <br> (h) I have three books.  These two are quite good, but this one is the *best* (book) *of all.* | Typical completions when a superlative is used: <br> In (f): *superlative* + *in a place* (*the world, this class, my family, the company, etc.*) <br><br> In (g): *superlative* + *adjective clause\** <br> In (h): *superlative* + **of all** |
| (i) Ali is *one of* the best *students* in this class. <br> (j) *One of* the best *students* in this class *is* Ali. | Note the pattern with **one of**: <br>   **one of** + *superlative* + *plural noun* <br> **One of** can also begin a sentence, as in (j). <br> NOTE:  A singular verb is used with **one of**. |

*See Chapter 12 for more information about adjective clauses.

**EXERCISE 15 ▸ Looking at grammar.  (Chart 9-3)**
Complete the sentences.  Use pronouns in the completions.

My Neighbors

1. Mr. Hanson is younger than his wife.  He's five years younger than ____*she is*____ OR
   (informally) ____*her*____ .

2. Mrs. Hanson works full-time.  Mr. Hanson works part-time.  She is busier than _____ .

3. Twins Marta and Mira are shy.  Their friends are more talkative than _____ .

4. Isabel's school is difficult, but mine is easy.  Isabel's school is more difficult than
   _____ .  My school is easier than _____ .

5. The Lees' house is big.  Our house is smaller than _____ .  Theirs is bigger than _____ .

6. My dad and I like to work on cars in our free time.  We are good mechanics, but Mr. Lu is a
   professional mechanic.  He is more knowledgeable about cars than _____ .

**EXERCISE 16 ▸ Looking at grammar.** (Chart 9-3)
Complete the sentences with superlatives of the words in *italics* and the preposition *in* or *of*,
where appropriate.

My English Class

1. Ken is *lazy.* He is _____*the laziest*_____ student ____*in*____ the class.

2. Phillip and Julia were *nervous,* but Erika was ____*the most nervous of all*____ .

3. Lucy doesn't need to study. She is naturally *smart.* She is one of _____
   students I have ever met.

4. Majda got a *bad* score on the test. It was one of _____ scores
   _____ the class.

5. There are a lot of *good* speakers in our class, but Daniel gives _____
   speeches _____ all.

6. Our teacher is very *kind.* She is one of _____ teachers I have ever met.

7. Our classroom is always *hot* and *uncomfortable.* It is one of _____ and
   _____ classrooms _____ the building.

8. Everyone was *exhausted* after the final exam, but I was _____ all.

**EXERCISE 17 ▸ Looking at grammar.** (Chart 9-3)
Complete the sentences with the superlative form of the words in *italics.*

1. I have had many *good experiences.* Of those, my vacation to Honduras was one of _____
   _____ I have ever had.

2. Ayako has had many *nice times,* but her birthday party was one of _____
   _____ she has ever had.

3. I've taken many *difficult courses,* but statistics is one of _____
   _____ I've ever taken.

4. I've made some *bad mistakes* in my life, but lending money to my cousin was one of _____
   _____ I've ever made.

5. We've seen many *beautiful buildings* in the world, but the Taj Mahal is one of _____
   _____ I've ever seen.

6. The *final exam* I took was pretty *easy.* In fact, it was one of _____
   _____ I've ever taken.

## EXERCISE 18 ▸ Let's talk: pairwork. (Chart 9-3)

Work with a partner. Take turns asking and answering questions. Use superlatives in your answers. Pay special attention to the use of plural nouns after *one of*.

*Example:*

PARTNER A: You have known many interesting people. Who is one of them?
PARTNER B: *One of* **the most interesting people** I've ever known *is* (\_\_\_\_). OR
(\_\_\_\_) **is** *one of* **the most interesting people** I've ever known.

1. There are many beautiful countries in the world. What is one of them?
2. There are many famous people in the world. Who is one of them?
3. You've probably seen many good movies. What is one of them?
4. You've probably done many interesting things in your life. What is one of them?
5. Think of some happy days in your life. What was one of them?
6. There are a lot of interesting animals in the world. What is one of them?
7. You have probably had many good experiences. What is one of them?
8. You probably know several funny people. Who is one of them?

## EXERCISE 19 ▸ Game. (Charts 9-1 → 9-3)

Work in teams. Compare each list of items using the words in *italics*. Write sentences using the comparative (*-er/more*) and the superlative (*-est/most/one of the*). The group with the most correct sentences wins.

*Example:*   streets in this city: *wide / narrow / busy / dangerous*
→ *First Avenue is* **wider** *than Market Street (is).*
→ *First Avenue is* **narrower** *than Interstate Highway 70.*
→ **The busiest** *street is Main Street.*
→ *Main Street is* **busier** *than Market Street.*
→ *Olive Boulevard is* **one of the busiest** *streets in the city.*
→ **The most dangerous** *street in the city is Olive Boulevard.*

1. a lemon, a grapefruit, and an orange:  *sweet / sour / large / small*

_____

_____

2. a kitten, a cheetah, and a lion:  *weak / powerful / wild / gentle / fast*

_____

_____

3. boxing, soccer, and golf:  *dangerous / safe / exciting / boring*

_____

_____

4. the food at (*three places in this city where you have eaten*):  *delicious / appetizing / inexpensive / good / bad*

_____

_____

**EXERCISE 20 ▸ Looking at grammar.** (Charts 9-1 → 9-3)
Complete the sentences with any appropriate form of the words in parentheses. Add any other necessary words.

Interesting Facts

1. Diamonds are very hard. They are (*hard*) _____*harder than*_____ rocks.
   They are one of (*hard*) _____*the hardest*_____ materials ___*of*___ all.

2. Crocodiles and alligators are different. The snout of a crocodile is (*long*)
   _____ and (*narrow*) _____ than an alligator's
   snout. An alligator has a (*wide*) _____ upper jaw than a
   crocodile.

3. The Great Wall of China is (*long*) _____
   structure that a country has ever built.

4. World Cup Soccer is (*big*) _____ sporting event
   _____ the world.

5. Young people have (*high*) _____ rate of car accidents
   _____ all drivers.

6. No animals can travel (*fast*) _____ than birds. Birds are (*fast*)
   _____ animals of all.

7. Bears are fast runners. Bears can run (*quick*) _____ than humans. Among
   bears, humans, and horses, bears can run short distances (*quick*)
   _____ of all.

8. One of (*active*) _____ volcanoes
   _____ the world is Mount Kilauea in Hawaii.

9. It's possible that the volcanic explosion of Krakatoa near Java in 1883 was
   (*loud*) _____ noise _____ recorded history.
   People heard it 2,760 miles/4,441 kilometers away.

**EXERCISE 21 ▸ Warm-up.** (Chart 9-4)
Complete the sentences with the names of people you know. Make true statements.

1. I speak English more slowly than _____.

2. I read English faster than _____.

## 9-4 Making Comparisons with Adverbs

|  |  |
|---|---|
| V    ADV<br>(a) Ryan runs *slowly*.<br>(b) Ryan runs *more slowly than* Tim.<br>(c) Ryan runs *the most slowly* of all his friends.<br>(d) Tim runs *faster than* Ryan. He runs *the fastest* of all his friends. | Adverbs modify verbs. Most adverbs end in *-ly*.<br>Adverbs can be used in comparisons, as in (b)–(d).<br>NOTE: The comparative and superlative forms of some adverbs like **fast** and **hard** do not end in *-ly*, as in (d). |
| (e) He works harder *than I do*.<br>(f) I arrived earlier *than they did*. | Frequently an auxiliary verb follows the subject after **than**.<br>In (e): *than I do = than I work*<br>In (f): *than they did = than they arrived* |

|  | ADVERB | COMPARATIVE | SUPERLATIVE |  |
|---|---|---|---|---|
| -LY ADVERBS | carefully<br>slowly | **more carefully**<br>**more slowly** | **the most carefully**<br>**the most slowly** | **More** and **most** are used with adverbs that end in *-ly*.* |
| ONE-SYLLABLE<br>ADVERBS | fast<br>hard | **faster**<br>**harder** | **the fastest**<br>**the hardest** | The *-er* and *-est* forms are used with one-syllable adverbs. |
| IRREGULAR<br>ADVERBS | well<br>badly<br>far | **better**<br>**worse**<br>**farther/further** | **the best**<br>**the worst**<br>**the farthest/the furthest** | Both **farther** and **further** are used to compare physical distances: *I walked farther than my friend did.* OR *I walked further than my friend did.* As an adjective, **further** also means "additional": *I need further information.*<br><br>Note that **farther** cannot be used when the meaning is "additional." |

*Exception: **early** is both an adjective and an adverb. Forms: *earlier, earliest.*

## EXERCISE 22 ▸ Looking at grammar. (Chart 9-4)
Complete the sentences with the correct form of the adverbs in parentheses.

**My Teachers**

1. Professor Gomez speaks (*quick*) _____*quickly*_____.

2. Professor Gomez speaks (*quick*) _____*more quickly*_____ than Professor Thom.

3. Professor Thom writes the answers (*slow*) _____ on the board.

4. My writing teacher corrects our essays (*careful*) _____.

5. My writing teacher correct our essays (*careful*) _____ than the other writing teachers.

6. Dr. Gupta comes to school at 6:00 A.M.  He comes (*early*) _____ than the director of the school.

7. Dr. Gupta comes to school (*early*) _____ of all the teachers.

8. Ms. Lee works (*hard*) _____ every day.

9. Ms. Lee works (*hard*) _____ than any other teacher I have.

10. Ms. Lee works (*hard*) _____ of all.

## EXERCISE 23 ▶ Looking at grammar.  (Charts 9-1 → 9-4)
Complete each sentence with the correct form of an adjective or adverb in the box.  Use each choice only once.

| careful | more careful | more carefully | the most careful | the most carefully |

1. Patrick drives _____ than his friends.

2. Patrick is a _____ driver.

3. Patrick is _____ driver of all his friends.

4. Patrick is a _____ driver than his friends.

5. Patrick drives _____ of all his friends.

| quick | quicker | more quickly | the quickest | the most quickly |

6. Andrea is a _____ runner.

7. Andrea runs _____ of all the members on her team.

8. Andrea runs _____ than the members on her team.

9. Andrea is a _____ runner than her friends.

10. Andrea is _____ runner of all her friends.

## EXERCISE 24 ▶ Looking at grammar. (Chart 9-4)

Choose the correct completions for each sentence. In some cases, both answers are correct.

1. Ron and his friend went jogging. Ron ran two miles, but his friend got tired after one mile. Ron ran _____ than his friend did.
   (a.) farther      (b.) further

2. If you have any _____ questions, don't hesitate to ask.
   a. farther      b. further

3. I gave my old computer to my younger sister because I had no _____ use for it.
   a. farther      b. further

4. Paris is _____ north than Tokyo.
   a. farther      b. further

5. I like my new apartment, but it is _____ away from school than my old apartment was.
   a. farther      b. further

6. Thank you for your help, but I'll be fine now. I don't want to cause you any _____ trouble.
   a. farther      b. further

7. Which is _____ from here: the subway or the train station?
   a. farther      b. further

## EXERCISE 25 ▶ Warm-up. (Chart 9-5)

Do you agree or disagree with these statements? Choose *yes* or *no*.

1. The grammar in this book is getting harder and harder.       yes     no

2. My English is getting better and better.       yes     no

3. The longer I study English, the better I get.       yes     no

| 9-5 | Repeating a Comparative; Using Double Comparatives | |
|---|---|---|
| (a) | Because he was afraid, he walked *faster and faster*. <br> (b) Life in the modern world is getting *more and more complicated*. | Repeating a comparative gives the idea that something becomes progressively greater, i.e., that it increases in intensity, quality, or quantity. |
| (c) | *The harder* you study, *the more* you will learn. <br> (d) *The more* she studied, *the more* she learned. <br> (e) *The warmer* the weather (is), *the better* I like it. | A double comparative has two parts; both parts begin with *the,* as in the examples. The second part of the comparison is the *result* of the first part. <br><br> In (c): If you study harder, the *result* will be that you will learn more. |
| (f) | — Do you want to ask Jenny and Jim to the party too? <br> — Why not? *The more, the merrier.* <br> (g) — When should we leave? <br> — *The sooner, the better.* | ***The more, the merrier*** and **the sooner, the better** are two common expressions. <br><br> In (f): It is good to have more people at the party. <br> In (g): We should leave as soon as we can. |

**EXERCISE 26 ▸ Looking at grammar.** (Chart 9-5)
Complete the sentences by repeating a comparative. Use the words in the box.

| | | | | |
|---|---|---|---|---|
| big | ✓ fast | hard | long | tired |
| discouraged | good | hot | loud | wet |

1. When I get nervous, my heart beats ____*faster and faster*____.

2. When you blow up a balloon, it gets _____
   _____.

3. Brian's health is improving. It's getting _____
   _____ every day.

4. As the ambulance came closer to us, the siren became _____
   _____.

5. The line of people waiting to get into the theater got _____
   _____ until it went around the building.

6. I've been looking for a job for a month and still haven't been able to find one.
   I'm getting _____.

7. As we traveled south toward the equator, the weather got _____
   _____.

8. The rain started as soon as I left my office. As I walked to the bus stop,
   it rained _____, and I got _____
   _____.

9. I tried to run up the steep hill, but my legs got _____,
   so I walked for a while.

**EXERCISE 27 ▸ Looking at grammar.** (Chart 9-5)
**Part I.** Complete the sentences with double comparatives (*the more/-er ... the more/-er*) and the words in *italics*.

1. If the fruit is *fresh*, it tastes *good*.

   ____*The fresher*____ the fruit (is), ____*the better*____ it tastes.

2. We got *close* to the fire. We felt *warm*.

   _____ we got to the fire, _____ we felt.

3. If a knife is *sharp*, it is *easy* to cut something with.

   _____ a knife (is), _____ it is to cut something.

4. The party got *noisy* next door. I got *angry*.

_____ it got, _____ I got.

5. I exercise for a *long* time. I get *thirsty*.

_____ I exercise, _____ I get.

**Part II.** Combine each pair of sentences. Use double comparatives (***the more/-er ... the more/-er***) and the words in *italics*.

6. Rosa offered to take me to the airport, and I was grateful. But we got a late start, so she began to drive faster.

She drove *fast*. \ I became *nervous*.

   *The faster she drove, the more nervous I became.*

7. Pierre tried to concentrate on his studies, but he kept thinking about his family and home.

He *thought* about his family. \ He became *homesick*.

_____

8. A storm was coming. We needed to get home.

The sky grew *dark*. \ We ran *fast*.

_____

## EXERCISE 28 ▸ Warm-up. (Chart 9-6)
Do you agree or disagree with these statements? Choose *yes* or *no*.

| | | |
|---|---|---|
| 1. I enjoy very cold weather. | yes | no |
| 2. It's a little cooler today than yesterday. | yes | no |
| 3. It's much warmer today than yesterday. | yes | no |

### 9-6 Modifying Comparatives with Adjectives and Adverbs

| | |
|---|---|
| (a) Tom is *very* old.<br>(b) Ann drives *very* carefully. | ***Very*** often modifies adjectives, as in (a), and adverbs, as in (b). |
| (c) INCORRECT: *Tom is very older than I am.*<br>    INCORRECT: *Ann drives very more carefully than she used to.* | ***Very*** is NOT used to modify comparative adjectives and adverbs. |
| (d) Tom is *much / a lot / far* older than I am.<br>(e) Ann drives *much / a lot / far* more carefully than she used to. | ***Much*, *a lot*,** or ***far*** are used to modify comparative adjectives and adverbs, as in (d) and (e). |
| (f) Ben is *a little (bit)* older than I am OR (*informally*) me. | Another common modifier is ***a little/a little bit***, as in (f). |

**EXERCISE 29 ▸ Looking at grammar. (Chart 9-6)**
Add *very*, *much*, *a lot*, or *far* to the sentences.

1. a. It's hot today. → It's **very** hot today.

   b. It's hotter today than yesterday. → It's **much** / **a lot** / **far** hotter today than yesterday.

2. a. An airplane is fast.

   b. Taking an airplane is faster than driving.

3. a. Learning a second language is difficult for many people.

   b. Learning a second language is more difficult than learning chemistry formulas.

4. a. You can live more inexpensively in student housing than in a rented apartment.

   b. You can live inexpensively in student housing.

**EXERCISE 30 ▸ Warm-up. (Chart 9-7)**
Which sentence matches this meaning? *The food is very spicy.*

   a. I've never tasted spicier food.

   b. I've never tasted spicy food.

| 9-7 Negative Comparisons | |
|---|---|
| (a) I've *never* taken a *harder* test. <br> (b) I've *never* taken a *hard* test. | **Never** + comparative = superlative <br> Example (a) means "It was the hardest test I've ever taken. I've never taken a harder test than this." Compare (a) and (b). |

**EXERCISE 31 ▸ Grammar and listening. (Chart 9-7)**
**Part I.** Choose the sentence (a. or b.) that is closest in meaning to the given sentence.

1. I've never been on a bumpier plane ride.
   a. The flight was very bumpy.          b. The flight wasn't bumpy.

2. I've never tasted hot chili peppers.
   a. The peppers are hot.          b. I haven't eaten hot chili peppers.

3. The house has never looked cleaner.
   a. The house looks very clean.          b. The house doesn't look clean.

4. We've never visited a more beautiful city.
   a. The city was beautiful.          b. The city wasn't beautiful.

 **Part II.** Listen to the sentences. Choose the sentence (a. or b.) that is closest in meaning to the one you hear.

5. a. His jokes are funny.          b. His jokes aren't funny.

6. a. It tastes great.          b. It doesn't taste very good.

7. a. The mattress is hard.          b. I haven't slept on hard mattresses.

8. a. The movie was very scary.          b. I haven't watched scary movies.

## EXERCISE 32 ▶ Warm-up. (Chart 9-8)

Compare the lengths of the lines.

1. Line D is as long as Line _____ .

2. Line A isn't as long as Line _____ .

3. Line E is almost as long as Line _____ .

Line A _____

Line B _____

Line C _____

Line D _____

Line E _____

## 9-8 Using As … As to Make Comparisons

| | |
|---|---|
| (a) Niki is 19 years old. Emilio is also 19. Niki is *as old as* Emilio (is). | *As … as* is used to say that the two parts of a comparison are equal or the same in some way. In (a): *as* + *adjective* + *as* |
| (b) Mike came *as quickly as* he could. | In (b): *as* + *adverb* + *as* |
| (c) Alex is 17. Niki is 19. Alex is *not as old as* Niki. (d) Alex is *not quite as old as* Niki. (e) Maya is 45. Alex is *not nearly as old as* Maya. | Negative form: *not as … as.** *Quite* and *nearly* are often used with the negative. In (d): *not quite as … as* = a small difference In (e): *not nearly as … as* = a big difference |
| (f) Niki is *just as old as* Emilio. (g) Alex is *nearly/almost As old as* Emilio. | Common modifiers of *as … as* are *just* (meaning "exactly") and *nearly/almost*. |

Niki
19

Alex
17

Emilio
19

Maya
45

*Also possible: *not so … as:* *Alex is *not so old as* Niki.*

## EXERCISE 33 ▶ Looking at grammar. (Chart 9-8)

Complete the sentences with *just as*, *almost as*, *not quite as*, or *not nearly as*. Answers may vary.

**Part I.** Compare the fullness of the glasses.

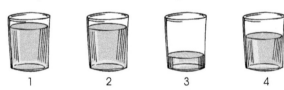

1    2    3    4

1. Glass 4 is _____ *almost as / not quite as* _____ full as Glass 2.

2. Glass 3 is _____ full as Glass 2.

3. Glass 1 is _____ full as Glass 2.

**Part II.** Compare the size of the boxes.

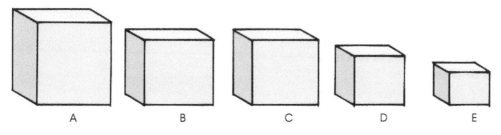

A       B       C       D       E

4. Box B is _____ big as Box A.

5. Box E is _____ big as Box A.

6. Box C is _____ big as Box B.

7. Box E is _____ big as Box D.

**EXERCISE 34 ▶ Looking at grammar.** (Chart 9-8)
Complete the sentences with **as ... as** and words in the box or your own words. Give your own opinion. Use negative verbs where appropriate.

| | |
|---|---|
| ✓ a housefly / an ant | good health / money |
| a lake / an ocean | honey / sugar |
| a lemon / a lime | monkeys / people |
| ✓ a lion / a tiger | physics / computer science |
| a shower / a bath | reading a book / watching a movie |
| a speck of sand / a speck of dust | the sun / the moon |

1. _An ant isn't as_ _____ big as _a housefly_ _____ .

2. _A lion is as_ _____ dangerous and wild as _a tiger_ _____ .

3. _____ large as _____ .

4. _____ sweet as _____ .

5. _____ important as _____ .

6. _____ sour as _____ .

7. _____ hot as _____ .

8. _____ good at climbing trees as _____ .

9. _____ relaxing as _____ .

10. _____ as tiny as _____ .

11. _____ as entertaining as _____ .

12. _____ as difficult as _____ .

**EXERCISE 35 ▶ Let's talk: pairwork.** (Chart 9-8)

Work with a partner. Take turns comparing the people in the photos. Use *as ... as* or *not as ... as*. You can also use *quite*, *almost*, and *nearly*. Your sentences can be true or false. Say your sentence to your partner. Your partner will answer *True* or *False*.

*Example:* PARTNER A: Amira is as old as Tia.
PARTNER B: False.

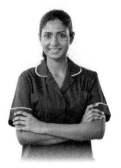

Tia, 30

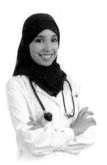

Amira, 28

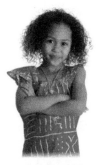

Jasmine, 10

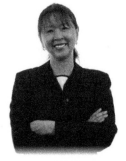

Sachi, 50

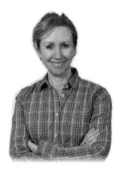

Emily, 50

**EXERCISE 36 ▶ Game.** (Chart 9-8)

*As ... as* is used in many traditional phrases. These phrases are generally spoken rather than written. See how many of them you're familiar with by completing the sentences with the given words. Work in teams. The team with the most correct answers wins.

| | | | | |
|---|---|---|---|---|
| ✓ a bear | a cat | a hornet | a mule | an ox |
| a bird | a feather | a kite | a rock | the hills |

1. When will dinner be ready? I'm **as** hungry **as** ____*a bear*____ .

2. Did Toshi really lift that heavy box all by himself? He must be **as** strong **as**

   _____ .

3. It was a lovely summer day. School was out, and there was nothing in particular that I

   had to do. I felt **as** free **as** _____ .

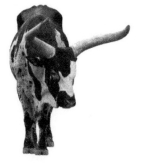

an ox

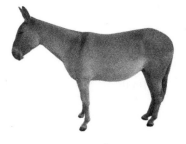

a mule

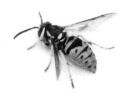

a hornet

4. Marco won't change his mind. He's **as** stubborn **as** _____.

5. How can anyone expect me to sleep in this bed? It's **as** hard **as** _____.

6. Of course I've heard that joke before! It's **as** old **as** _____.

7. Why are you walking back and forth? What's the matter? You're **as** nervous **as**

_____.

8. Thanks for offering to help, but I can carry the box alone. It looks heavy, but it isn't. It's **as** light **as** _____.

9. When Erica received the good news, she felt **as** high **as** _____.

10. A: Was he angry?

B: You'd better believe it! He was **as** mad **as** _____.

## EXERCISE 37 ▸ Listening. (Charts 9-1 → 9-3, 9-7, and 9-8)
Listen to each sentence and choose the statement (a. or b.) that has a similar meaning.

*Example:*  You will hear:     I need help! Please come as soon as possible.
            You will choose:   ⓐ Please come quickly.
                               b. Please come when you have time.

1. a. Business is better this year.
   b. Business is worse this year.

2. a. Steven is a very friendly person.
   b. Steven is an unfriendly person.

3. a. The test was difficult for Sam.
   b. The test wasn't so difficult for Sam.

4. a. We can go farther.
   b. We can't go farther.

5. a. Jon made a very good decision.
   b. Jon made a very bad decision.

6. a. I'm going to drive faster.
   b. I'm not going to drive faster.

7. a. Your work was careful.
   b. Your work was not careful.

8. a. I'm not hungry.
   b. I would like to eat.

9. a. My drive and my flight take the same amount of time.
   b. My drive takes more time.

## EXERCISE 38 ▸ Warm-up. (Chart 9-9)

Complete the sentences with your own words.

1. Compare the cost of two cars:

   (*A/An*) _____ is more expensive than (*a/an*) _____ .

2. Compare the cost of two kinds of fruit:

   _____ are less expensive than _____ .

3. Compare the cost of two kinds of shoes (boots, sandals, tennis shoes, flip-flops, etc.):

   _____ are not as expensive as _____ .

4. Compare the cost of two kinds of heat:  (gas, electric, solar, wood, coal, etc.):

   _____ is not as cheap as _____ .

| 9-9 | Using *Less ... Than* and *Not As ... As* | |
|---|---|---|
| MORE THAN ONE SYLLABLE:<br>(a)  A pen is *less expensive than* a book.<br><br>(b)  A pen is *not as expensive as* a book. | The opposite of **-er/more** is expressed by **less** or **not as ... as**.<br><br>Examples (a) and (b) have the same meaning. | |
| | **Less** and **not as** ... **as** are used with adjectives and adverbs of *more than one syllable*. | |
| ONE SYLLABLE:<br>(c)  A pen is *not as large as* a book.<br>      INCORRECT:  *A pen is less large than a book.* | Only **not as ... as** (NOT **less**) is used with *one-syllable adjectives or adverbs*, as in (c). | |

## EXERCISE 39 ▸ Looking at grammar.  (Chart 9-9)

Choose the correct completions for each sentence. In some cases, both answers are correct.

1. My nephew is _____ old _____ my niece.
   - a. less ... than
   - b. not as ... as

2. My nephew is _____ hard-working _____ my niece.
   - a. less ... than
   - b. not as ... as

3. A bee is _____ big _____ a bird.
   - a. less ... than
   - b. not as ... as

4. My brother is _____ interested in computers _____ I am.
   - a. less ... than
   - b. not as ... as

5. Some students are _____ serious about their schoolwork _____ others.
   - a. less ... than
   - b. not as ... as

6. I am _____ good at repairing things _____ Diane is.
   - a. less ... than
   - b. not as ... as

**EXERCISE 40 ▸ Game.** (Charts 9-1 → 9-3 and 9-7 → 9-9)

Work in teams. Compare the given words using (*not*) *as ... as*, *less*, and *more/-er*. How many comparison sentences can you think of? The team with the most correct sentences wins.

*Example:* trees and flowers (*big, colorful, useful, etc.*)
→ *Trees are bigger than flowers.*
→ *Flowers are usually more colorful than trees.*
→ *Flowers are less useful than trees.*
→ *Flowers aren't as tall as trees.*

1. the sun and the moon
2. teenagers and adults
3. two restaurants in this area
4. two famous people in the world

**EXERCISE 41 ▸ Listening.** (Charts 9-1, 9-8, and 9-9)

Listen to each sentence and the statements that follow it. Choose "T" for true or "F" for false.

*Examples:* France \ Brazil
You will hear: a. France isn't as large as Brazil.
You will choose: (T)   F

You will hear: b. France is bigger than Brazil.
You will choose: T   (F)

1. a sidewalk \ a road
   a.  T    F
   b.  T    F

2. a hill \ a mountain
   a.  T    F
   b.  T    F

3. hiking along a mountain path \ climbing a mountain peak
   a.  T    F
   b.  T    F

4. toes \ fingers
   a.  T    F
   b.  T    F
   c.  T    F

5. basic math \ algebra
   a.  T    F
   b.  T    F
   c.  T    F
   d.  T    F

**EXERCISE 42 ▸ Warm-up: trivia.** (Chart 9-10)

Compare Manila, Seattle, and Singapore. Which two cities have more rain in December?*

_____ and _____ have more rain than

_____ in December.

*See *Trivia Answers*, p. 443.

## 9-10 Using *More* with Nouns

| | |
|---|---|
| (a) Would you like some *more coffee*? <br> (b) Not everyone is here. I expect *more people* to come later. | In (a): **Coffee** is a noun. When **more** is used with nouns, it often has the meaning of "additional." It is not necessary to use **than**. |
| (c) There are *more people* in China *than* there are in Canada. | **More** is also used with nouns to make complete comparisons by adding **than**. |
| (d) Do you have enough coffee, or would you like some *more*? | When the meaning is clear, the noun may be omitted and **more** can be used by itself. |

**EXERCISE 43 ▶ Looking at grammar.** (Charts 9-1, 9-4, and 9-10)
Use the words in the box to complete the sentences. Add **more** as necessary.

| | | | |
|---|---|---|---|
| cheap | cleaner | noisier | safer |
| cheaper | ✓ money | noisy | safely |
| cheaply | noise | pollution | traffic |

Country Life

1. Prices are lower outside the city, and I'm saving _____*more money*_____ than I did in the city.

2. The city was expensive. I'm living _____ in the country than in the city.

3. Apartments are _____ in the country than in the city.

4. It took me only a day to find a comfortable and _____ apartment.

5. I didn't drive in the city. There were so many cars. A city has _____ than a small town.

6. I used to take the bus and subway, but now I drive a lot on two-lane highways. I have to be careful and drive _____ because I don't want to have an accident.

7. There is less crime in my town. Life is _____ for me in the country than in the city.

8. The air is very clean in my town. The city has more _____ than the country.

9. The air in the country is _____ than the air in the city.

10. The city was very loud. I heard traffic all day long. There is _____ in the city than in the country.

11. I didn't sleep well at night. Ambulances often woke me up. The city is _____ than the country.

12. I'm glad to live in a quiet area. The city was a very _____ place for me.

**EXERCISE 44 ▸ Game: trivia.** (Chart 9-10)
Work in teams. Write true sentences using the given information. The team with the most correct sentences wins.*

1. more kinds of mammals: South Africa \ Kenya
   → *Kenya has more kinds of mammals than South Africa.*
2. more volcanoes: Indonesia \ Japan
3. more moons: Saturn \ Venus
4. more people: Saõ Paulo, Brazil \ New York City
5. more islands: Greece \ Finland
6. more mountains: Switzerland \ Nepal
7. more sugar (per 100 grams): an apple \ a banana
8. more fat (per 100 grams): the dark meat of a chicken \ the white meat of a chicken

**EXERCISE 45 ▸ Warm-up.** (Chart 9-11)
Solve the math problems and then complete the sentences. Some answers may vary.

PROBLEM A:   $2 + 2 =$
PROBLEM B:   $\sqrt{900} + 20 =$
PROBLEM C:   $3 \times 127 =$
PROBLEM D:   $2 + 3 =$
PROBLEM E:   $127 \times 3 =$

1. Problem _____ and Problem _____ have the same answers.

2. Problem _____ and Problem _____ have similar answers.

3. Problem _____ and Problem _____ have different answers.

4. The answer to Problem _____ is the same as the answer to Problem _____.

5. The answers to Problem _____ and Problem _____ are similar.

6. The answers to Problem _____ Problem _____ are different.

7. Problem _____ has the same answer as Problem _____.

8. Problem _____ is like Problem _____.

9. Problem _____ and Problem _____ are alike.

---

*See *Trivia Answers*, p. 443.

## 9-11 Using *The Same, Similar, Different, Like, Alike*

| | |
|---|---|
| (a) Paul and Mia have *the same books*.<br>(b) Paul and Mia have *similar books*.<br>(c) Paul and Mia have *different books*.<br>(d) Their books are *the same*.<br>(e) Their books are *similar*.<br>(f) Their books are *different*. | *The same*, *similar*, and *different* are used as adjectives.<br><br>NOTE: *the* always precedes *same*. |
| (g) This book is *the same as* that one.<br>(h) This book is *similar to* that one.<br>(i) This book is *different from* that one. | NOTE: *the same* is followed by *as*;<br>　　　*similar* is followed by *to*;<br>　　　*different* is followed by *from*.* |
| (j) She is *the same age as* my mother.<br>　　My shoes are *the same size as* yours. | A noun may come between *the same* and *as*, as in (j). |
| (k) My pen *is like* your pen.<br>(l) My pen *and* your pen *are alike*. | Note in (k) and (l):<br><br>　*noun + be like + noun*<br>　*noun and noun + be alike* |
| (m) She *looks like* her sister.<br>　　It *looks like* rain.<br>　　It *sounds like* thunder.<br>　　This material *feels like* silk.<br>　　That *smells like* gas.<br>　　This chemical *tastes like* salt.<br>　　Stop *acting like* a fool.<br>　　He *seems like* a nice guy. | In addition to following *be*, *like* also follows certain verbs, primarily those dealing with the senses.<br><br>Note the examples in (m). |
| (n) The twins *look alike*.<br>　　We *think alike*.<br>　　Most four-year-olds *act alike*.<br>　　My sister and I *talk alike*.<br>　　The little boys are *dressed alike*. | *Alike* may follow a few verbs other than *be*.<br><br>Note the examples in (n). |

*In informal speech, native speakers might use *than* instead of *from* after *different*. *From* is considered correct in formal English, unless the comparison is completed by a clause: *I have a different attitude now than I used to have.*

## EXERCISE 46 ▶ Looking at grammar. (Chart 9-11)

Complete the sentences with *as, to, from*, or *Ø*.

1. a. Geese are similar _to_ ducks. They are both large water birds.

   b. But geese are not the same _____ ducks. Geese are usually
   
   larger and have longer necks.

   c. Geese are different _____ ducks.

   d. Geese are like _____ ducks in some ways, but geese and ducks
   
   are not exactly alike _____ .

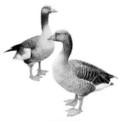

geese

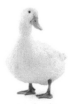

a duck

an orange · a peach

2. a. An orange is not the same _____ a peach.

   b. An orange is like _____ a peach in some ways, but they are not exactly

      alike _____ .

   c. An orange is similar _____ a peach. They are both round, sweet, and juicy.

   d. An orange is different _____ a peach.

## EXERCISE 47 ▶ Looking at grammar. (Chart 9-11)

Compare the diagrams. Complete the sentences with *the same* (*as*), *similar* (*to*), *different* (*from*), *like*, or *alike*. Answers may vary.

1. All of the diagrams are ____*similar to*____ each other.

2. A is _____ B.

3. A and B are _____ .

4. A and C are _____ .

5. A and C are _____ D.

6. C is _____ A.

7. B isn't _____ D.

A          B

C          D

## EXERCISE 48 ▶ Grammar and listening. (Charts 9-1 and 9-11)

Complete the sentences with the words in the box. Then listen to each passage and correct your answers.

| | | | |
|---|---|---|---|
| alike | from | more | the |
| as | like | than | to |

Gold vs. Silver

Gold is similar _____ silver. They are both valuable
                          1

metals that people use for jewelry, but they aren't _____ same.
                                                        2

Gold is not _____ same color _____ silver. Gold is
                3                              4

also different _____ silver in cost: gold is _____ expensive
                  5                                        6

_____ silver.
      7

Do you know these words?
- metals        - stripes
- valuable      - unique
- pattern

**Two Zebras**

Look at the two zebras in the picture. Their names are Zee and

Bee. Zee looks _____ Bee. Is Zee exactly _____
              1                                              2

same _____ Bee? The pattern of the stripes on each zebra
            3

in the world is unique. No two zebras are exactly _____ .
                                                         4

Even though Zee and Bee are similar _____ each other, they are
                                                  5

different _____ each other in the exact pattern of their stripes.
                6

## EXERCISE 49 ▶ Looking at grammar. (Chart 9-11)

Complete the sentences with **the same (as)**, **similar (to)**, **different (from)**, **like**, or **alike**. In some cases, more than one completion may be possible.

1. Jennifer and Jack both come from Rapid City. In other words, they come from

   _____*the same*_____ town.

2. This city is ____*the same as / similar to / like*____ my hometown. Both are quiet and conservative.

3. You and I don't agree. Your ideas are _____ mine.

4. Sergio never wears _____ clothes two days in a row.

5. A male mosquito is not _____ size _____ a female mosquito. The female is larger.

6. I'm used to stronger coffee. I think the coffee at this cafe tastes _____ dishwater.

7. *Meet* and *meat* are homonyms; in other words, they have _____ pronunciation.

8. *Flower* has _____ pronunciation _____ *flour*.

9. My twin sisters act _____, but they don't look _____ .

10. Trying to get through school without studying is _____ trying to go swimming without getting wet.

## EXERCISE 50 ▶ Check your knowledge. (Chapter 9 Review)

Correct the errors in comparison structures.

1. Did you notice? My shoes and your shoes are a̶ *the* same.

2. Alaska is largest state in the United States.

3. A pillow is soft, more than a rock.

4. Who is most generous person in your family?

5. The harder you work, you will be more successful.

6. One of a biggest disappointment in my life was when my soccer team lost the championship.

7. My sister is very more talkative than I am.

8. A firm mattress is so comfortable for many people than a soft mattress.

9. One of the most talkative student in the class is Frederick.

10. Professor Bennett's lectures were the confusingest I have ever heard.

**EXERCISE 51 ▶ Reading.** (Chapter 9 Review)
**Part I.** Read the passage and the statements that follow it.
Underline five comparative or superlative structures.
NOTE: *He* and *she* are used interchangeably.

Do you know these words?
- influence          - turn out to be
- personality        - artistic
- characteristics    - creative
- somewhat           - self-centered
- get along with     - raise
- peacekeeper

# BIRTH ORDER

In your family, are you the oldest, youngest, middle, or only child? Some psychologists believe your place in the family, or your birth order, has a strong influence on your personality. Let's look at some of the personality characteristics of each child.

The oldest child has all the parents' attention when she is born. As she grows up, she may want to be the center of attention. Because she is around adults, she might act more like an adult around other children and be somewhat controlling. As the oldest, she might have to take care of the younger children, so she may be more responsible. She may want to be the leader when she is in groups.

The middle child (or children) may feel a little lost. Middle children have to share their parents' attention. They may try to be different from the oldest child. If the oldest child is "good," the second child may be "bad." However, since they need to get along with both the older and younger sibling(s), they may be the peacekeepers of the family.

The youngest child is the "baby" of the family. Other family members may see him as weaker, smaller, or more helpless. If the parents know this is their last child, they may not want the child to grow up as quickly as the other children. As a way to get attention, the youngest child may be the funniest child in the family. He may also have more freedom and turn out to be more artistic and creative.

An only child (no brothers or sisters) often grows up in an adult world. Such children may use adult language and prefer adult company. Only children may be more intelligent and more serious than other children their age. They might also be more self-centered because of all the attention they get, and they might have trouble sharing with others.

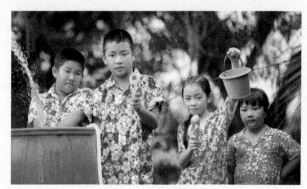

Of course, these are general statements. A lot depends on how the parents raise the child, how many years are between each child, and the culture the child grows up in. How about you? Do you see any similarities to your family?

**Part II.** Read the statements. Circle "T" for true and "F" for false according to the information in the passage.

1. The two most similar children are the oldest and only child.          T          F

2. The middle child often wants to be like the oldest child.          T          F

3. The youngest child likes to control others.          T          F

4. Only children may want to spend more time with adults.          T          F

5. All cultures share the same birth order characteristics.          T          F

## EXERCISE 52 ▸ Writing. (Chapter 9)

**Part I.** Look at the list of adjectives that describe personality characteristics. Check (✓) the words you know. Then work with a partner. Ask your partner about the words you don't know. If neither of you knows, you can look them up.

| | | |
|---|---|---|
| artistic | funny | rebellious |
| competitive | hard-working | relaxed |
| controlling | immature | secretive |
| cooperative | loud | sensitive |
| creative | mature | serious |
| flexible | outgoing | shy |

**Part II.** Read the paragraph. <u>Underline</u> the comparative structures.

**My Father and I**

I am different from my father in several ways. He is more hard-working than I am. He is a construction worker and has to be at work at 6:00 A.M. He often doesn't get home until late in the evening. I'm a student, and I don't work as hard. I have much more free time, especially in the mornings and evenings. Another difference is that I am funnier than he is. I like to tell jokes and make people laugh. He is more serious, but he laughs at my jokes. My father was an athlete when he was my age, and he played a lot of team sports. Also, he is very competitive. I am not as competitive, and I don't like playing team sports. However, we like to watch them together on TV. My father and I are different from each other, but we like to spend time with each other. Our differences make our time together interesting.

**Part III.** Write a paragraph comparing your personality to that of another member of your family or a friend. Follow these steps:

1. Write an introductory sentence: *I am different from / similar to my ....*
2. Choose at least four characteristics from the word list. For each one, write a comparison. Use these structures:
   - *different from / (not) the same as / similar to*
   - *-er / more ... than*
   - *(not) as ... as*
3. Write a few details that explain each comparison.
4. Write a concluding sentence.

---

**WRITING TIP**

Transitional words like *but, however,* and *also* can help you to connect your comparative sentences better. These words make it easier for the reader to follow your ideas. *But* and *however* have the same meaning; *however* is a little more formal.

- He is more serious, but he laughs at my jokes.
- However, we like to watch them together on TV.

If you want to talk about a new difference or similarity, *another* is a useful word: *Another difference is...* or *Another similarity is....*

- Another difference is that I am funnier than he is.

Look at the paragraph again, and underline the words that help connect the ideas.

---

**Part IV.** Edit your writing. Check for the following:

1. ☐ correct use of comparative and superlative adjectives and adverbs (*-er/est* or *more/the most*)
2. ☐ correct prepositions with these phrases: *the same as/different from/similar to*
3. ☐ correct use of *as ... as* (no *than*)
4. ☐ use of some words to help connect your ideas, such as *but, however, also, another*
5. ☐ correct spelling (use a dictionary or spell-check)

---

▨▨▨▨▨ For digital resources, go to the Pearson Practice English app.

# CHAPTER 1

# The Passive

**PRETEST: What do I already know?**
Write "C" if the **boldfaced** words are correct and "I" if they are incorrect.

1. _____ Books **written** by authors.  (Charts 10-1 and 10-2)

2. _____ The patient **is being seen** by Dr. Vinh.  (Chart 10-3)

3. _____ The bus driver **was died** in the accident.  (Chart 10-4)

4. _____ What **was happened**?  (Chart 10-4)

5. _____ My watch **was made** in China.  (Chart 10-5)

6. _____ Your passport **must be checked** by the customs officer.  (Chart 10-6)

7. _____ Michael **is married to** Helena.  (Chart 10-7)

8. _____ Water **is composed oxygen** and hydrogen.  (Chart 10-7)

9. _____ I have a headache.  The lecture was so **bored**.  (Chart 10-8)

10. _____ Rika **got** really **nervous** before her final exam.  (Chart 10-9)

11. _____ We **are not accustomed to live** in a small town.  (Chart 10-10)

12. _____ I **am used to sleeping** on a hard mattress.  (Chart 10-11)

13. _____ You **supposed to** be home before midnight.  (Chart 10-12)

**EXERCISE 1 ▶ Warm-up.  (Charts 10-1 and 10-2)**
Choose the sentence in each pair that describes the picture above it.  More than one answer
may be correct.

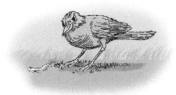

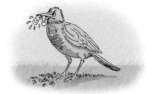

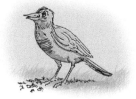

1. a. The worm is watching
      the bird.

   b. The bird is watching
      the worm.

2. a. The bird caught the
      worm.

   b. The worm was caught
      by the bird.

3. a. The bird ate the worm.

   b. The worm was eaten.

## 10-1 Active and Passive Sentences

| | |
|---|---|
| **Active**<br>(a) The mouse *ate* the cheese.<br><br>**Passive**<br>(b) The cheese *was eaten* by the mouse. | Examples (a) and (b) have the same meaning. |

| **Active** | **Passive** |
|---|---|
| 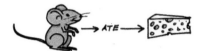 | 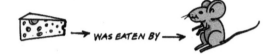 |

| | |
|---|---|
| **Active**<br>s            o<br>(c) Bob     mailed     the package.<br>**Passive**<br>s           by + o<br>(d) The package   was mailed   by Bob. | Sentence (c) is an active sentence: *Bob* is the subject and *the package* is the object.<br><br>Sentence (d) is a passive sentence. The object of the active sentence becomes the subject. The subject of the active sentence is the object of **by**. |

## 10-2 Forming the Passive

| | | | | |
|---|---|---|---|---|
| | *BE* | + | PAST PARTICIPLE | |
| (a) Corn | *is* | | *grown* | by farmers. |
| (b) The fish | *was* | | *caught* | by Ava. |

Form of all passive verbs: **be** + *past participle*

**Be** can be in any of its forms: *am, is, are, was, were, has been, have been, will be, etc.*

| | Active | Passive |
|---|---|---|
| SIMPLE PRESENT | Farmers *grow* corn. ⟶ | Corn *is grown* by farmers. |
| SIMPLE PAST | Farmers *grew* corn. ⟶ | Corn *was grown* by farmers. |
| PRESENT PERFECT | Farmers *have grown* corn. ⟶ | Corn *has been grown* by farmers. |
| FUTURE | Farmers *will grow* corn. ⟶ | Corn *will be grown* by farmers. |
| | Farmers *are going to grow* corn. ⟶ | Corn *is going to be grown* by farmers. |

## EXERCISE 2 ▸ Looking at grammar. (Charts 10-1 and 10-2)

Write the **be** verb and the past participle if a sentence has them.
Then write "P" if the sentence is passive.

**At the Dentist**

|     |                                                      | **BE** | **+** | **PAST PARTICIPLE** |     |
| --- | ---------------------------------------------------- | ------ | ----- | ------------------- | --- |
| 1.  | The dentist checks your teeth.                       | Ø      |       | Ø                   |     |
| 2.  | Your teeth are checked by the dentist.               | *are*  |       | *checked*           | P   |
| 3.  | The dental assistant cleaned your teeth.             |        |       |                     |     |
| 4.  | Your teeth were cleaned by the dental assistant.     |        |       |                     |     |
| 5.  | You have a cavity.                                   |        |       |                     |     |
| 6.  | You are going to need a filling.                     |        |       |                     |     |
| 7.  | Fillings are done by the dentist.                    |        |       |                     |     |
| 8.  | You will need to schedule another appointment.       |        |       |                     |     |
| 9.  | Another appointment will be needed.                  |        |       |                     |     |

## EXERCISE 3 ▸ Looking at grammar. (Charts 10-1 and 10-2)

Who does what? Work in pairs. Complete the sentences with the simple present form of the passive
and the correct word in the box.

| authors | construction workers | pharmacists | plumbers |
| --- | --- | --- | --- |
| ✓auto mechanics | firefighters | pilots | vets/veterinarians |

1. Cars (*repair*) _____are repaired_____ by _____auto mechanics_____ .
2. Toilets (*fix*) _____ by _____ .
3. Planes (*fly*) _____ by _____ .
4. Fires (*fight*) _____ by _____ .
5. Animals (*treat*) _____ by _____ .
6. Books (*write*) _____ by _____ .
7. Buildings (*build*) _____ by _____ .
8. Prescriptions (*fill*) _____ by _____ .

## EXERCISE 4 ▸ Looking at grammar. (Charts 10-1 and 10-2)

Change the active verbs to passive by adding the correct subjects and forms of **be**.

1. **SIMPLE PRESENT**

   a. The teacher *helps* **me**.   ___I___ ___am_____ **helped** by the teacher.

   b. The teacher *helps* **Eva**.   ___Eva___ ___is_____ **helped** by the teacher.

   c. The teacher *helps* **us**.   _____ _____ **helped** by the teacher.

2. **SIMPLE PAST**

    a. The teacher *helped* **him**.   _____ _____ **helped** by the teacher.

    b. The teacher *helped* **them**.   _____ _____ **helped** by the teacher.

3. **PRESENT PERFECT**

    a. The teacher *has helped* **her**.   _____ _____ **helped** by the teacher.

    b. The teacher *has helped* **Joe**.   _____ _____ **helped** by the teacher.

4. **FUTURE**

    a. The teacher *will help* **me**.   _____ _____ **helped** by the teacher.

    b. The teacher *is going to help* **us**. _____ _____ **helped** by the teacher.

## EXERCISE 5 ▸ Looking at grammar. (Charts 10-1 and 10-2)

Change the verbs from active to passive. Do not change the tenses.

Tech Tasks

|  |  | BE | + | PAST PARTICIPLE |  |
|---|---|---|---|---|---|
| 1. Leo *scanned* the photos. | The photos | *were* | | *scanned* | by Leo. |
| 2. A team *edits* the documents. | The documents | _____ | | _____ | by a team. |
| 3. An assistant *has changed* the passwords. | The passwords | _____ | | _____ | by an assistant. |
| 4. Mari *is going to upload* a video. | The video | _____ | | _____ | by Mari. |
| 5. A secretary *will delete* files. | Files | _____ | | _____ | by a secretary. |
| 6. Tim *fixed* the printer. | The printer | _____ | | _____ | by Tim. |

## EXERCISE 6 ▸ Looking at grammar. (Charts 10-1 and 10-2)

Complete the sentences with the correct passive form of the verb.

In the News

1. The town is going to offer free Wi-Fi.

    Free Wi-Fi _____ by the town.

2. The police took the suspect to jail.

    The suspect _____ to jail by the police.

3. Government officials pay their taxes late.

    Taxes _____ late by government officials.

4. The city has designed a new park.

A new park _____ by the city.

5. Our football team will win the championship.

The championship _____ by our football team.

## EXERCISE 7 ▶ Looking at grammar. (Charts 10-1 and 10-2)
Choose the sentences that are logical (make sense).

Laws of Nature

1. (a.) Big fish eat little fish.
   (b.) Little fish are eaten by big fish.
   c. Little fish eat big fish.

2. a. Bees make honey.
   b. Honey makes bees.
   c. Honey is made by bees.

3. a. Mice hunt cats.
   b. Mice are hunted by cats.
   c. Cats are hunted by mice.
   d. Cats hunt mice.

4. a. The earth heats the sun.
   b. The earth is heated by the sun.
   c. The sun heats the earth.

5. a. Lightning hits people.
   b. People are hit by lightning.
   c. People hit lightning.
   d. Lightning is hit by people.

6. a. Humans eat animals.
   b. Animals are eaten by humans.
   c. Animals eat humans.
   d. Humans are eaten by animals.

## EXERCISE 8 ▶ Looking at grammar. (Charts 10-1 and 10-2)
Change the sentences from active to passive.

A Graduation Party

| ACTIVE | PASSIVE |
|---|---|
| 1. a. The party will surprise Sam. | *Sam will be surprised by the party* . |
| b. Will the party surprise Max? | *Will Max be surprised by the party* ? |
| 2. a. Ana planned the party. | _____ . |
| b. Did Ari plan the party too? | _____ ? |
| 3. a. Greta will order food. | _____ . |
| b. Will Pat order food too? | _____ ? |
| 4. a. Jill is going to sign the card. | _____ . |
| b. Is Ryan going to sign it? | _____ ? |
| 5. a. Joni has made decorations. | _____ . |
| b. Has Kazu made decorations? | _____ ? |

**EXERCISE 9 ▸ Looking at grammar.** (Charts 10-1 and 10-2)
Which sentences express the meaning of the given sentence? More than one answer may be possible.

At School

1. A teacher interviewed the students for the scholarship.
   a. The students were interviewed.
   b. Someone interviewed the students.
   c. The teacher was interviewed.

2. Ms. Kinea was asked to teach a photography class.
   a. Ms. Kinea asked to teach photography.
   b. Someone asked Ms. Kinea to teach photography.
   c. Ms. Kinea asked someone to teach photography.

3. The students are told to clean the classrooms at the end of the day.
   a. The students told people to clean the classrooms.
   b. The classrooms are cleaned by the students.
   c. Someone told the students to clean the classrooms.

4. The staff checks student IDs.
   a. Someone checks student IDs.
   b. Student IDs are checked by someone.
   c. The staff is checked.

5. The principal will choose the graduation speakers soon.
   a. The graduation speakers will be chosen soon.
   b. The graduation speakers will choose soon.
   c. The principal will be chosen soon.

**EXERCISE 10 ▸ Warm-up.** (Chart 10-3)
Check (✓) the actions that are or were in progress.

1. _____ The fish are being fed by the boy.

2. _____ The fish were fed by the boy.

3. _____ The fish were being fed by the boy.

4. _____ The boy is feeding the fish.

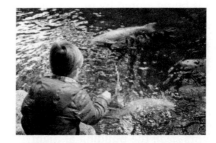

| **10-3** Progressive Forms of the Passive | | |
|---|---|---|
| | **Active** | **Passive** |
| PRESENT PROGRESSIVE | Lyn *is copying* the files. ⟶ | The files *are being copied* by Lyn. |
| PAST PROGRESSIVE | Lyn *was copying* the files. ⟶ | The files *were being copied* by Lyn. |

# EXERCISE 11 ▸ Looking at grammar. (Chart 10-3)

Change the active verbs to passive by adding the correct form of **be**. Include the subject of the passive sentence.

1. **PRESENT PROGRESSIVE**

   a. A tutor *is helping* **us.** _____ _____ **helped** by a tutor.

   b. A tutor *is helping* **her.** _____ _____ **helped** by a tutor.

   c. A tutor *is helping* **me.** _____ _____ **helped** by a tutor.

   d. A tutor *is helping* **them.** _____ _____ **helped** by a tutor.

2. **PAST PROGRESSIVE**

   a. A tutor *was helping* **me.** _____ _____ **helped** by a tutor.

   b. A tutor *was helping* **him.** _____ _____ **helped** by a tutor.

   c. A tutor *was helping* **us.** _____ _____ **helped** by a tutor.

   d. A tutor *was helping* **you.** _____ _____ **helped** by a tutor.

# EXERCISE 12 ▸ Looking at grammar. (Chart 10-3)

Change each sentence from passive to active.

A Company Video

1. The script was being written by professional writers.
   → *Professional writers were writing the script.*
2. Music is being chosen by a producer.
3. Subtitles are being written by a manager.
4. The film is being edited by the director.
5. Photos were being added by an assistant.

# EXERCISE 13 ▸ Looking at grammar. (Charts 10-1 → 10-3)

Complete the verbs.

An Office Building at Night

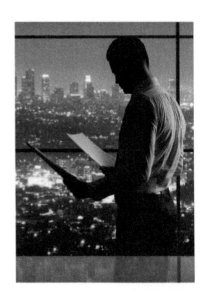

1. The janitors *clean* the building at night.

   The building ___*is*___ clean*ed*_____ by the janitors at night.

2. Janitors *clean* the carpets.

   The carpets _____ clean_____ by janitors.

3. The owner *is reviewing the* rents.

   Rents _____ review_____ by the

   owner.

4. The owner *is going to announce* rent increases.

Rent increases _____ announce_____ by the owner.

5. An electrician *is fixing* some lights.

Some lights _____ fix_____ by an electrician.

6. The security guard *has checked* the offices.

The offices _____ check_____ by the security guard.

7. The security guard *discovered* an open window.

An open window _____ discover_____ by the security guard.

8. The security guard *found* an unlocked door.

An unlocked door _____ found by the security guard.

## EXERCISE 14 ▶ Looking at grammar. (Charts 10-1 → 10-3)

Change these questions from active to passive.

Hotel Questions

1. Has the maid cleaned our room yet?
   → *Has our room been cleaned by the maid yet?*
2. Does the hotel provide hair dryers?
3. Did housekeeping bring extra towels?
4. Has room service brought our meal?
5. Is the bellhop* bringing our luggage to our room?
6. Is maintenance going to fix the air-conditioning?
7. Will the front desk upgrade** our room?

## EXERCISE 15 ▶ Warm-up. (Chart 10-4)

Check (✓) the sentences that have objects. <u>Underline</u> the objects.

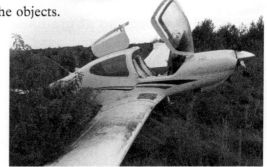

1. _____ A small plane crashed.
2. _____ The plane hit a tree.
3. _____ The tree fell on the wing.
4. _____ Fortunately, the pilot didn't die.
5. _____ The crash didn't kill the pilot.

---

*bellhop* = a person who carries luggage for hotel guests

**upgrade* = make better; in this case, provide a better room than the original one. *Upgrade* is a regular verb.

## 10-4 Transitive and Intransitive Verbs

| **Transitive** | | | A TRANSITIVE verb has an object. An object is a noun or a pronoun. |
|---|---|---|---|
| s | v | o | |
| (a) Alan | wrote | the song. | |
| (b) Mr. Lee | signed | the check. | |
| (c) A cat | killed | the bird. | |

| **Intransitive** | | | An INTRANSITIVE verb does NOT have an object. |
|---|---|---|---|
| s | v | | |
| (d) Something | happened. | | |
| (e) Kate | came | to our house. | NOTE: *to our house* is a prepositional phrase. It is not the object of the verb *came*. See Chart 6-4, p. 164. |
| (f) The bird | died. | | |

| **Transitive Verbs** | | Only transitive verbs can be used in the passive. |
|---|---|---|
| (g) ACTIVE: | Alan *wrote* the song. | |
| (h) PASSIVE: | The song *was written* by Alan. | |

| **Intransitive Verbs** | | An intransitive verb is NOT used in the passive. |
|---|---|---|
| (i) ACTIVE: | Something *happened*. | |
| (j) PASSIVE: | *(not possible)* | |
| (k) INCORRECT: | *Something was happened.* | |

**Common Intransitive Verbs***

| | | | | |
|---|---|---|---|---|
| agree | die | happen | rise | stand |
| appear | exist | laugh | seem | stay |
| arrive | fall | live | sit | talk |
| become | flow | occur | sleep | wait |
| come | go | rain | sneeze | walk |

*To find out if a verb is transitive or intransitive, look in your dictionary. The usual abbreviations are v.t. (transitive) and v.i. (intransitive). Some verbs have both transitive and intransitive uses. For example:
  transitive: *Students study books.*
  intransitive: *Students study.*

## EXERCISE 16 ▶ Looking at grammar. (Chart 10-4)

Check (✓) the sentences that have an object. <u>Underline</u> the objects.

1. a. _____ Jimmy sold his car.

   b. _____ Jimmy drove a truck to work.

   c. _____ Jimmy drove in a truck to work.

2. a. _____ Mr. Ortiz died at home at midnight.

   b. _____ A heart attack killed him.

3. a. _____ We arrived late to the wedding.

   b. _____ We came to the wedding in a taxi.

4. a. _____ Something strange happened at school today.

   b. _____ A car went off the road.

   c. _____ It hit a tree near a classroom.

**EXERCISE 17 ▶ Looking at grammar.** (Chart 10-4)
Underline the verbs and identify them as transitive (v.t.) or intransitive (v.i.).
If possible, change the sentences to the passive.

1. Omar <u>walked</u> to school yesterday. *(no change)*  [v.i.]

2. Alexa <u>broke</u> the window. → *The window was broken by Alexa.*  [v.t.]

3. The leaves fell to the ground.

4. I slept at my friend's house last night.

5. Many people felt an earthquake yesterday.

6. Dinosaurs existed millions of years ago.

7. I usually agree with my sister.

8. Many people die during a war.

9. Scientists will discover a cure for cancer someday.

10. Did the Italians invent spaghetti?

**EXERCISE 18 ▶ Game: trivia.** (Charts 10-1 → 10-4)
Work in teams. Make true statements. Match the information in the left column with the
information in the right column. Some sentences are active and some are passive. Add ***was/were***
as necessary. The team with the most correct answers (facts and grammar) wins.★

*Examples:* 1. Alexander Eiffel __h__. *(no change)*
2. Anwar Sadat __c__. → *Anwar Sadat was shot in 1981.*

1. Alexander Eiffel __h__.

2. Anwar Sadat __c__.

3. Princess Diana _____.

4. Marie and Pierre Curie _____.

5. Oil _____.

6. Nelson Mandela _____.

7. Michael Jackson _____.

8. Leonardo da Vinci _____.

9. John F. Kennedy _____.

10. Romeo and Juliet _____.

a. killed in a car crash in 1997

b. died in 2009

✓ c. shot in 1981

d. painted the *Mona Lisa*

e. elected president of the
United States in 1960

f. discovered in Saudi Arabia in 1938

g. kept apart by their parents

✓ h. designed the Eiffel Tower

i. released from prison in 1990

j. discovered radium

---

★See *Trivia Answers*, p. 443.

**EXERCISE 19 ▸ Warm-up.** (Chart 10-5)

Complete the sentences with information from one of your textbooks.

1. _____ was written by _____.
   (name of book)

2. It was published by _____.

| 10-5 | Using the *by*-Phrase |
| --- | --- |

| | |
| --- | --- |
| (a) This sweater *was made* **by my aunt**. | The *by*-phrase is used in passive sentences when it is important to know who performs an action.<br><br>In (a): **by my aunt** is important information. |
| (b) My sweater *was made* in Korea.<br>(c) Spanish *is spoken* in Colombia.<br>(d) That house *was built* in 1900.<br>(e) Rice *is grown* in many countries. | Usually there is no *by*-phrase in a passive sentence.<br><br>The passive is used when it is *not known or not important to know exactly who performs an action*.<br><br>In (b): The exact person (or people) who made the sweater is not known and is not important to know, so there is no *by*-phrase in the passive sentence. |
| (f) *My aunt* is very creative. *She made* this sweater.<br>(g) A: I like your sweaters.<br>B: Thanks. *This sweater was made by* my aunt. *That sweater was made by* my mother. | Usually the active is used when the speaker knows who performed the action, as in (f), where the focus of attention is on **my aunt**.<br><br>In (g): Speaker B uses the passive with a *by*-phrase because he wants to focus attention on the subjects of the sentences. The focus of attention is on the two sweaters. The *by*-phrases add important information. |

**EXERCISE 20 ▸ Looking at grammar.** (Chart 10-5)

Both a. and b. sentences are grammatically correct. Choose the better sentence in each pair.

The Taj Mahal

1. Workers began construction of the Taj Mahal in 1632.
   a. Construction of the Taj Mahal was begun in 1632.
   b. Construction of the Taj Mahal was begun in 1632 by workers.

2. About 22,000 workers, artists, and craftsmen built the Taj Mahal.
   a. The Taj Mahal was built.
   b. The Taj Mahal was built by about 22,000 workers, artists, and craftsmen.

3. Builders built the Taj Mahal with materials from all over Asia.
   a. The Taj Mahal was built with materials from all over Asia.
   b. The Taj Mahal was built with materials from all over Asia by builders.

4. More than 1,000 elephants delivered the building materials to the site.
   a. The building materials were delivered to the site.
   b. The building materials were delivered to the site by more than 1,000 elephants.

5. Decorators decorated some of the walls with gemstones.
   a. Some of the walls were decorated with gemstones.
   b. Some of the walls were decorated with gemstones by decorators.

**EXERCISE 21 ▶ Looking at grammar.** (Chart 10-5)
Change the sentences from active to passive. Include the *by*-phrase only as necessary.

Around the World

1. People grow rice in India. _____ *Rice is grown in India.* _____

2. Do people grow rice in Africa? _____

3. People speak Portuguese in Brazil. _____

4. Canadians speak French. _____

5. Where do people speak Spanish? _____

6. Alibaba® and Amazon® sell online products. _____

7. People eat junk food in every country. _____

**EXERCISE 22 ▶ Looking at grammar.** (Charts 10-1 → 10-5)
Make sentences with the given words. Some sentences are active and some are passive.

At a Pizza Restaurant

1. The dough \ make \ by the owner

   a. (*every day*) _____ *The dough is made by the owner every day.* _____

   b. (*yesterday*) _____

   c. (*tomorrow*) _____

2. The owner \ make \ the dough

   a. (*every week*) _____

   b. (*last week*) _____

3. The sauce \ prepare \ by his wife

   a. (*right now*) _____

   b. (*every day*) _____

   c. (*tomorrow*) _____

4. His wife \ prepare \ the sauce

   a. (*in the mornings*) _____

   b. (*a few minutes ago*) _____

5. The dough \ throw \ up in the air

   a. (*now*) _____

   b. (*in a few minutes*) _____

6. Pizzas \ bake \ in a pizza oven

   a. (*now*) _____

   b. (*all day long yesterday*) _____

   c. (*recently*) _____

## EXERCISE 23 ▸ Looking at grammar. (Charts 10-1 → 10-5)

Make sentences with the given words, either orally or in writing. Some sentences are active and some are passive. Use the past tense. Do not change the order of the words.

### A Traffic Stop

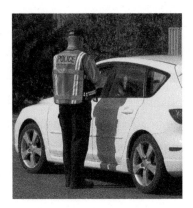

1. The police \ stop \ a speeding car
   → *The police stopped a speeding car.*
2. The driver \ ask \ to get out of the car \ by the police
3. The driver \ take out \ his license
4. The driver \ give \ his license \ to the police officer
5. The license \ check
6. The driver \ give \ a ticket
7. The driver \ tell \ to drive more carefully

 ## EXERCISE 24 ▸ Grammar and listening. (Charts 10-1 → 10-5)

Listen to the passage. Listen again and complete the sentences with the verbs you hear.

### A Bike Accident

A: Did you hear about the accident outside the dorm entrance?

B: No. What _____1_____?

A: A guy on a bike _____2_____ by a taxi.

B: _____3_____ he _____4_____?

A: Yeah. Someone _____5_____ an ambulance.

He _____6_____ to

City Hospital and _____7_____

in the emergency room for cuts and bruises.

B: What _____8_____ to the taxi driver?

A: He _____9_____ for reckless driving.

B: He's lucky that the bicyclist _____10_____.

> Do you know these words?
> - dorm
> - guy
> - treated
> - bruises
> - arrest
> - reckless
> - bicyclist

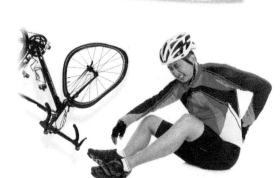

## EXERCISE 25 ▸ Looking at grammar. (Charts 10-1 → 10-5)

Complete the sentences with the correct form (active or passive) of the verbs in parentheses.

1. Yesterday our teacher (*arrive*) _____*arrived*_____ five minutes late.
2. Last night class (*cancel*) _____ because of snow.
3. That's not my coat. It (*belong*) _____ to Lara.
4. Our mail (*deliver*) _____ before noon every day.

5. The "b" in *comb* (*pronounce, not*) _____ . It is silent.

6. What (*happen*) _____ to John? Where is he?

7. When I (*arrive*) _____ at the airport yesterday, I (*meet*)
_____ by my cousin and a couple of her friends.

8. Yesterday Lee and I (*hear*) _____ about Scott's divorce. I (*surprise, not*)
_____ by the news, but Lee (*shock*)
_____ .

9. A new house (*build*) _____ next to ours next year.

10. Roberto (*send*) _____ that message last week. This one (*send*)
_____ yesterday.

11. At the soccer game yesterday, the winning goal (*kick*) _____ by Luigi.
Over 100,000 people (*attend*) _____ the soccer game.

12. A: I think American football is too violent.

B: I (*agree*) _____ with you. I (*prefer*) _____ baseball.

13. A: When (*your bike, steal*) _____ ?

B: Two days ago.

14. A: (*you, pay*) _____ your electric bill yet?

B: No, I haven't, but I'd better pay it today. If I don't, my electricity (*shut off*)
_____ by the power company.

## EXERCISE 26 ▶ Warm-up. (Chart 10-6)
Read the paragraph and then the statements. Circle "T" for true and "F" for false.

### Getting a Passport

Jerry is applying for a passport. He is going to fill out the application form online.
He needs to take his application, proof of citizenship, and two passport photos to the passport
office. He also has to pay a fee. He will receive his passport in the mail about three weeks after
he applies for it.

1. All of the steps for a passport can be done online.     T     F

2. Proof of citizenship must be provided.     T     F

3. A fee has to be paid.     T     F

4. Photographs should be taken after he applies.     T     F

5. The passport will be sent by mail.     T     F

## 10-6 Passive Modal Auxiliaries

| Active Modal Auxiliaries | Passive Modal Auxiliaries (*modal* + ***be*** + *past participle*) | | | Modal auxiliaries are often used in the passive. |
|---|---|---|---|---|
| Bob *will mail it.* | It | *will be mailed* | by Bob. | **FORM:** |
| Bob *can mail it.* | It | *can be mailed* | by Bob. | *modal* + ***be*** + *past participle* |
| Bob *should mail it.* | It | *should be mailed* | by Bob. | (See Chapter 7 for information about the |
| Bob *ought to mail it.* | It | *ought to be mailed* | by Bob. | meanings and uses of modal auxiliaries.) |
| Bob *must mail it.* | It | *must be mailed* | by Bob. | |
| Bob *has to mail it.* | It | *has to be mailed* | by Bob. | |
| Bob *may mail it.* | It | *may be mailed* | by Bob. | |
| Bob *might mail it.* | It | *might be mailed* | by Bob. | |
| Bob *could mail it.* | It | *could be mailed* | by Bob. | |

**EXERCISE 27 ▶ Looking at grammar.** (Chart 10-6)
Complete the sentences by changing the active modals to passive.

**Money Matters**

1. Someone must pay this bill immediately.
   This bill ____*must be paid*____ immediately.

2. The bank may request additional information.
   Additional information _____ by the bank.

3. People cannot avoid taxes.
   Taxes _____.

4. Someone has to pay credit card interest.
   Credit card interest _____.

5. People can reach the bank manager on his cell phone at 555-3815.
   The bank manager _____ on his cell phone at 555-3815.

6. The bank should issue* a refund.
   A refund _____ by the bank.

7. People may pay the amount now or later.
   The amount _____ now or later.

8. Be careful! If that bank app isn't secure, someone could steal your money.
   Your money _____ if that bank app isn't secure.

9. My parents say students must save money for college.
   My parents say money _____ for college.

---

*issue = give, provide

**EXERCISE 28 ▶ Reading and grammar.** (Charts 10-1 → 10-6)

Are you wearing jeans right now or do you have a pair at home? Who were they made by? Read the passage about jeans and choose the correct verbs.

# HOW JEANS WERE INVENTED

Around the world, a very popular pant for men, women, and children is jeans. Did you know that jeans created / were created more than 100 years ago?

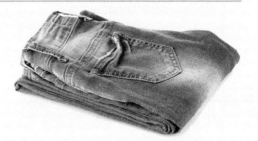

They invent / were invented by Levi Strauss during
the California Gold Rush.

In 1853, Levi Strauss, a 24-year-old immigrant from Germany, traveled / were travel from
New York to San Francisco. His brother was the owner of a store in New York and wanted to
open another one in San Francisco. When Strauss arrived / was arrived, a gold miner
asked / was asked him what he had to sell. Levi said he had strong canvas for tents and wagon
covers. The miner told him he really needed strong pants because he couldn't find any that
lasted very long.

So Levi Strauss took the canvas and designed / was designed a pair of overall pants.
The miners liked / were liked them except that they were rough on the skin. Strauss
changed / was changed the canvas to a cotton cloth from France called *serge de Nimes*.
Later, the fabric called / was called "denim" and the pants gave / were given the nickname
"blue jeans."

Eventually, Levi Strauss & Company formed / was formed. Strauss and tailor David Jacobs
began putting rivets in pants to make them stronger. In 1936, a red tab added / was added
to the rear pocket. This was done so "Levis" could identify / could be identified
more easily. Now the company is world famous. For many people, all jeans know / are known
as Levis.

# EXERCISE 29 ▸ Warm-up: trivia. (Chart 10-7)

Complete the sentences with words in the box.* Not all words are necessary.

| | | | |
|---|---|---|---|
| China | monkeys | sand | spiders |
| Mongolia | Nepal | small spaces | whales |

1. Glass is composed mainly of _____.

2. Dolphins are related to _____.

3. The Gobi Desert is located in two countries: _____ and _____.

4. People with claustrophobia are frightened of _____.

## 10-7 Past Participles as Adjectives (Stative or Non-Progressive Passive)

| | | | | |
|---|---|---|---|---|
| | BE | + | ADJECTIVE | Be can be followed by an adjective, as in (a)–(c). The adjective describes or gives information about the subject of the sentence. |
| (a) Paul | is | | young. | |
| (b) Paul | is | | tall. | |
| (c) Paul | is | | hungry. | |
| | BE | + | PAST PARTICIPLE | Be can be followed by a past participle (the passive form), as in (d)–(f). The past participle is often like an adjective. The past participle describes or gives information about the subject of the sentence. Past participles are used as adjectives in many common, everyday expressions. |
| (d) Paul | is | | married. | |
| (e) Paul | is | | tired. | |
| (f) Paul | is | | frightened. | |

| | |
|---|---|
| (g) Paul *is married to* Susan.<br>(h) Paul *was excited about* the game.<br>(i) Paul *will be prepared for* the exam. | Often the past participles in these expressions are followed by particular prepositions + an object. For example:<br> In (g): ***married*** is followed by ***to*** ( + *an object*)<br> In (h): ***excited*** is followed by ***about*** ( + *an object*)<br> In (i): ***prepared*** is followed by ***for*** ( + *an object*) |

**Expressions with *Be* + Past Participle and Common Prepositions**

| | | |
|---|---|---|
| be acquainted (*with*) | be excited (*about*) | be opposed (*to*) |
| be bored (*with, by*) | be exhausted (*from*) | be pleased (*with*) |
| be broken | be finished (*with*) | be prepared (*for*) |
| be closed | be frightened (*of*) | be qualified (*for*) |
| be composed of | be gone (*from*) | be related (*to*) |
| be crowded (*with*) | be hurt | be satisfied (*with*) |
| be devoted (*to*) | be interested (*in*) | be scared (*of*) |
| be disappointed (*in, with*) | be involved (*in, with*) | be shut |
| be divorced (*from*) | be located (*in, south of, etc.*) | be spoiled |
| be done (*with*) | be lost | be terrified (*of*) |
| be drunk (*on*) | be made of | be tired (*of, from*)* |
| be engaged (*to*) | be married (*to*) | be worried (*about*) |

*I'm **tired of** the cold weather. = I've had enough cold weather. I want the weather to get warm.
 I'm **tired from** working hard all day. = I'm tired because I worked hard all day.

*See Trivia Answers, p. 443.

## EXERCISE 30 ▸ Looking at grammar. (Chart 10-7)

Choose <u>all</u> the correct completions.

1. Roger is disappointed with _____ .
   a. his job
   b. in the morning
   c. his son's grades

2. Are you related to _____ ?
   a. the Browns
   b. math and science
   c. me

3. Finally! We are done with _____ .
   a. finished
   b. our chores
   c. our errands

4. My boss was pleased with _____ .
   a. my report
   b. thank you
   c. the new contract

5. The baby birds are gone from _____ .
   a. away
   b. their nest
   c. yesterday

6. Taka and Joanne are bored with _____ .
   a. their work
   b. this movie
   c. their marriage

7. Are you tired of _____ ?
   a. work
   b. asleep
   c. the news

## EXERCISE 31 ▸ Looking at grammar. (Chart 10-7)

**Part I.** Complete each sentence with an appropriate preposition.

*Nervous Nick is ...*

1. worried _____ almost everything in life.

2. frightened _____ being around people.

3. also scared _____ snakes, lizards, and dogs.

4. terrified _____ going outside and seeing a dog.

5. exhausted _____ worrying so much.

6. tired _____ his fears.

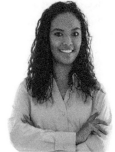

*Happy Halle is ...*

7. excited _____ waking up every morning.

8. pleased _____ her job.

9. interested _____ having a good time.

10. involved _____ many community activities.

11. satisfied _____ just about everything in her life.

12. qualified _____ a variety of jobs.

**Part II.** Work in small groups. Make three statements about yourself or someone in your family. Use the adjectives in Part I.

**EXERCISE 32 ▶ Looking at grammar.** (Chart 10-7)
Complete the sentences with a form of *be* + the past participle of the verbs in the box.
Note the prepositions in **bold** that follow them.

| | | | |
|---|---|---|---|
| compose | interest | oppose | satisfy |
| finish | marry | prepare | ✓scare |

1. Most young children _____ *are scared* _____ **of** loud noises.

2. Jane _____ **in** ecology.

3. Don't clear the table yet. I _____ not _____ **with** my meal.

4. I _____ **with** my progress in English.

5. Tony _____ **to** Sonia. They have a happy marriage.

6. Roberta's parents _____ **to** her marriage. They don't like her fiancé.

7. The test is tomorrow. _____ you _____ **for** it?

8. A digital picture _____ **of** thousands of tiny dots called pixels.

**EXERCISE 33 ▶ Looking at grammar.** (Chart 10-7)
Complete each sentence with an appropriate preposition.

1. Because of the sale, the mall was crowded _____ shoppers.

2. Do you think you are qualified _____ that job?

3. Mr. Ahmad loves his family very much. He is devoted _____ them.

4. My sister is married _____ a law student.

5. I'll be finished _____ my work in another minute or two.

6. The workers are opposed _____ the new health-care plan.

7. Are you acquainted _____ this writer? I can't put her books down!*

8. Janet doesn't take good care of herself. I'm worried _____ her health.

**EXERCISE 34 ▶ Let's talk.** (Chart 10-7)
Interview another student in the class. You will need to add prepositions to the questions.
Share a few of the answers with the class.

1. When will you be done _____ your English studies?

2. What are you excited _____ doing next year?

3. What are you not prepared _____ ?

4. Have you ever been involved _____ team sports? Where? When?

5. What do kids nowadays become bored _____ quickly?

6. Are you scared or terrified _____ anything? What?

---

*\*can't put a book down* = can't stop reading a book because it's so exciting/interesting

7. What are you opposed _____?

8. Are you related _____ anyone famous? Who?

## EXERCISE 35 ▶ Looking at grammar. (Chart 10-7)

Complete the sentences with the correct form of the expressions in the box.
Add prepositions as necessary.

| | | |
|---|---|---|
| be acquainted | be exhausted | be qualified |
| be composed | be located | be spoiled |
| be crowded | be made | ✓be worried |
| be disappointed | | |

1. Dennis isn't doing well in school this semester. He ___*is worried about*___ his grades.

2. My shirt _____ cotton.

3. I live in a small apartment with six people. Our apartment _____.

4. Vietnam _____ Southeast Asia.

5. I'm going to go straight to bed tonight. It's been a hard day. I _____.

6. The kids _____. I had promised to take them to the beach today, but now we can't go because it's raining.

7. Yuk! This milk tastes sour. I think it _____.

8. Water _____ hydrogen and oxygen.

9. The job description says an applicant must have a master's degree and five years of teaching experience. I _____ not _____ that job.

10. I've never met Mrs. Novinsky. I _____ not _____ her.

## EXERCISE 36 ▶ Listening. (Chart 10-7)

Complete the sentences with the words you hear.

*Example:* You will hear: My earrings are made of gold.
You will write: My earrings ___*are made of gold*___.

1. This fruit _____. I think I'd better throw it out.

2. When we got to the post office, it _____.

3. Oxford University _____ Oxford, England.

4. Haley doesn't like to ride in elevators. She's _____ small spaces.

5. What's the matter? _____ you _____?

6. Excuse me. Could you please tell me how to get to the bus station from here?
   I _____.

7. Your name is Tom Hood? _____ you _____ Mary Hood?

8. Where's my wallet? It's _____! Did someone take it?

9. Oh, no! Look at my sunglasses. I sat on them, and now they _____ .

10. It's starting to rain. _____ all of the windows _____?

## EXERCISE 37 ▸ Warm-up. (Chart 10-8)
Match the sentences with the pictures. Two sentences do not match either picture.

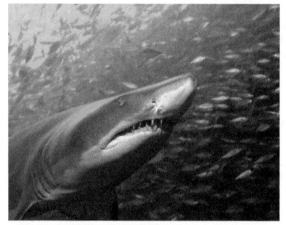
Picture A

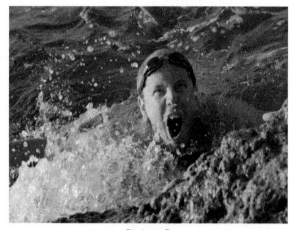
Picture B

1. The shark is terrifying. _____

2. The shark is terrified. _____

3. The swimmer is terrifying. _____

4. The swimmer is terrified. _____

---

### 10-8 Participial Adjectives: *-ed* vs. *-ing*

| | |
|---|---|
| Art **interests** me.<br><br>(a) I am *interested* in art.<br>    INCORRECT: *I am interesting in art.*<br><br>(b) Art is *interesting*.<br>    INCORRECT: *Art is interested.*<br><br>The news **surprised** Kate.<br>(c) Kate was *surprised*.<br>(d) The news was *surprising*. | The past participle (*-ed* )* and the present participle (*-ing*) can be used as adjectives.<br><br>In (a): The past participle (*interested*) describes how a person feels.<br><br>In (b): The present participle (*interesting*) describes the *cause* of the feeling. The cause of the interest is art.<br><br>In (c): ***surprised*** describes how Kate felt. The past participle carries a passive meaning: *Kate was surprised **by the news***.<br><br>In (d): ***the news*** was the cause of the surprise. |
| (e) Did you hear the *surprising news*?<br>(f) Dino fixed the *broken window*. | Like other adjectives, participial adjectives may follow ***be***, as in examples (a) through (d), or they may come in front of nouns, as in (e) and (f). |

*The past participle of regular verbs ends in *-ed*. For verbs that have irregular forms, see Chart 2-3, p. 33, Appendix A-2, and the inside back cover.

## EXERCISE 38 ▶ Looking at grammar. (Chart 10-8)

Make sentences about the pictures. Use *roller coaster*, *younger woman*, and *older woman*.

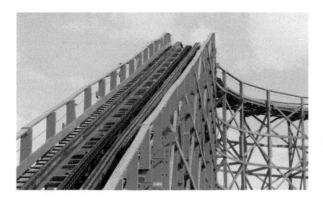
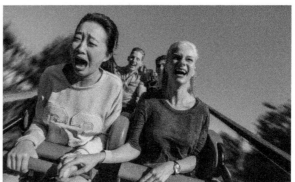

A Roller Coaster Ride

1. The _____ is frightened.

2. The _____ is frightening.

3. The _____ is excited.

4. The _____ is exciting.

5. The _____ is thrilling.

6. The _____ is delighted.

## EXERCISE 39 ▶ Looking at grammar. (Chart 10-8)

Complete the sentences with the *-ed* or *-ing* form of the verbs in *italics*.

1. Talal's classes *interest* him.

   a. Talal's classes are _____*interesting*_____ .

   b. Talal is an _____*interested*_____ student.

2. Emily is going to Australia. The idea of going on this trip *excites* her.

   a. Emily is _____ about going on this trip.

   b. She thinks it is going to be an _____ trip.

3. I like to study sea life. The subject of marine biology *fascinates* me.

   a. Marine biology is a _____ subject.

   b. I'm _____ by marine biology.

4. Mike heard some bad news. The bad news *depressed* him.

   a. Mike is very sad. In fact, he is _____ .

   b. The news made Mike feel very sad. The news was _____ .

5. Robots *interest* me.

   a. I'm _____ in robots.

   b. Robots are _____ to me.

## EXERCISE 40 ▸ Listening. (Chart 10-8)

Listen to the statements and choose the words you hear.

*Example:* You will hear: It was a frightening experience.

You will choose:  frighten  (frightening)  frightened

| | | |
|---|---|---|
| 1. bore | boring | bored |
| 2. shock | shocking | shocked |
| 3. confuse | confusing | confused |
| 4. embarrass | embarrassing | embarrassed |
| 5. surprise | surprising | surprised |
| 6. scare | scary* | scared |

## EXERCISE 41 ▸ Looking at grammar. (Chart 10-8)

Choose the correct word in each sentence.

SITUATION: Nicki was walking on the beach with her co-worker Tyler during their lunch break. She slipped on some rocks and fell into the water.

1. Nicki felt   embarrassed / embarrassing.

2. Falling into the water was   embarrassed / embarrassing for her.

3. It was an   embarrassed / embarrassing   experience.

4. Tyler was   surprised / surprising   when he heard the splash.

5. He had a   surprised / surprising   look on his face.

6. When Nicki went back to the office, her co-workers were   interested / interesting   in her story.

7. Nicki said her story wasn't   interesting / interested.

8. But weeks later, she could laugh about it. Now the story is   amused / amusing.

9. Nicki is   amused / amusing   when she thinks about the story.

## EXERCISE 42 ▸ Warm-up. (Chart 10-9)

Are these statements true for you? Circle *yes* or *no.*

*Right now ...*

| | | |
|---|---|---|
| 1. I am getting tired. | yes | no |
| 2. I am getting hungry. | yes | no |
| 3. I am getting confused. | yes | no |

---

*The adjective ending is **-y**, not **-ing**.

## 10-9 Get + Adjective; Get + Past Participle

| | |
|---|---|
| GET + ADJECTIVE<br><br>(a) I *am getting hungry*. Let's eat.<br><br>(b) Eric *got nervous* before the job interview. | **Get** can be followed by an adjective. **Get** gives the idea of change — the idea of becoming, beginning to be, growing to be.<br><br>In (a): **I'm getting hungry**. = *I wasn't hungry before, but now I'm beginning to be hungry.* |
| GET + PAST PARTICIPLE<br><br>(c) I'm *getting tired*. Let's stop working.<br><br>(d) Steve and Rita *got married* last month. | Sometimes **get** is followed by a past participle. The past participle after **get** is like an adjective; it describes the subject of the sentence. |

**Get + Adjective**

| | | |
|---|---|---|
| get angry | get dry | get quiet |
| get bald | get fat | get rich |
| get big | get full | get serious |
| get busy | get hot | get sick |
| get close | get hungry | get sleepy |
| get cold | get interested | get thirsty |
| get dark | get late | get well |
| get dirty | get nervous | get wet |
| get dizzy | get old | |

**Get + Past Participle**

| | | |
|---|---|---|
| get acquainted | get drunk | get involved |
| get arrested | get engaged | get killed |
| get bored | get excited | get lost |
| get confused | get finished | get married |
| get crowded | get frightened | get scared |
| get divorced | get hurt | get sunburned |
| get done | get interested | get tired |
| get dressed | get invited | get worried |

## EXERCISE 43 ▶ Looking at grammar. (Chart 10-9)

Complete the sentences with the words in the box.

| | | | | |
|---|---|---|---|---|
| bald | dirty | hurt | lost | rich |
| busy | ✓full | late | nervous | serious |

1. This food is delicious, but I can't eat any more. I'm getting ___*full*___.

2. Stop wasting time! We need to get _____ and finish our project!

3. I didn't understand Mariam's directions very well, so on the way to her house last night I got _____. I couldn't find her house.

4. It's hard to work on a car and stay clean. Paul's clothes always get _____ from all the grease and oil.

5. Tim doesn't like to fly. His heart beats quickly during takeoff. He gets _____.

6. We'd better go home. It's getting _____, and you have school tomorrow.

7. Simon wants to get _____, but he doesn't want to work. That's not very realistic.

8. If you plan to go to medical school, you need to get _____ about the time and money involved and start planning now.

9. Mr. Andersen is losing some of his hair. He's slowly getting _____.

10. Was the accident serious? Did anyone get _____?

## EXERCISE 44 ▸ Let's talk: interview. (Chart 10-9)

Interview your classmates. Share some of their answers with the class.

1. Have you ever gotten hurt? What happened?
2. Have you ever gotten lost? What happened?
3. When was the last time you got dizzy?
4. How long does it take you to get dressed in the morning?
5. In general, do you get sleepy during the day? When?
6. Do you ever get hungry in the middle of the night? What do you do?
7. Have you ever gotten involved with a charity? Which one?

## EXERCISE 45 ▸ Listening. (Chart 10-9)

Listen to the sentences and complete them with any adjectives that make sense.

***Example:*** You will hear: This towel is soaking wet. Please hang it up so it will get _____.

You will write: _____*dry*_____

1. _____   3. _____   5. _____

2. _____   4. _____   6. _____

## EXERCISE 46 ▸ Reading. (Chart 10-9)

Read the passage and the statements that follow it. Circle "T" for true and "F" for false.

**A Blended Family**

Lisa and Thomas live in a blended family. They are not related to each other, but they are brother and sister. Actually, they are stepbrother and stepsister. This is how they came to be in the same family.

Lisa's mother got divorced when Lisa was a baby. Thomas' father was a widower. His wife had died unexpectedly. Lisa and Thomas' parents met a few years ago at a going-away party for a friend. After a year of dating, they got engaged, and a year later, they got married. Lisa is older than Thomas, but they get along well. Theirs is a happy blended family.

> Do you know these words?
> - blend            - unexpectedly
> - related to       - dating
> - widower

1. Lisa's mother got married. Then she got divorced. Then she got remarried.   T  F

2. Thomas' father got married, and then he got divorced. After he got divorced, he got engaged, and then he got remarried.   T  F

3. Lisa and Thomas became stepsister and stepbrother when their parents got married.   T  F

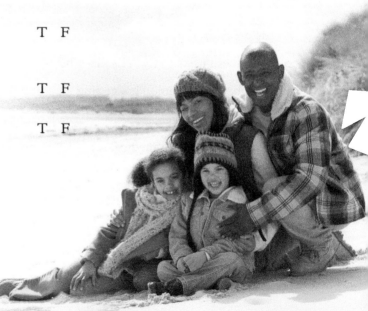

**EXERCISE 47 ▶ Looking at grammar.** (Chart 10-9)
Complete the sentences with appropriate forms of **get** and the words in the box.

| | | | | |
|---|---|---|---|---|
| angry | dark | hungry | lost | tired |
| cold | dressed | involve | marry | well |
| crowd | dry | kill | ✓sunburn | worry |

1. When I stayed out in the sun too long yesterday, I _____ _got sunburned_____ .

2. If you're sick, stay home and take care of yourself. You won't _____ if you don't take care of yourself.

3. Alima and Hasan are engaged. They are going to _____ a year from now.

4. Sarah doesn't eat breakfast, so she always _____ by ten or ten-thirty.

5. In the winter, the sun sets early. It _____ outside by six or even earlier.

6. Put these towels back in the dryer. They didn't _____ the first time.

7. Let's stop working for a while. I'm _____ . I need a break.

8. Anastasia has to move out of her apartment next week, and she hasn't found a new place to live.
   She's _____ .

9. Toshiro was in a terrible car wreck and almost _____ . He's lucky to be alive.

10. The temperature is dropping. Brrr! I'm _____ . Can I borrow your sweater?

11. Sorry we're late. We took a wrong turn and _____ .

12. Good restaurants _____ around dinner time. It's hard to find a seat because there are so many people.

13. Calm down! Take it easy! You shouldn't _____ so _____ . It's not good for your blood pressure.

14. I left when Ellen and Joe began to argue. I never _____ in other people's quarrels.

15. Sam is wearing one brown sock and one blue sock today. He _____ in a hurry this morning and didn't pay attention to the color of his socks.

**EXERCISE 48 ▶ Warm-up.** (Chart 10-10)
Circle the words in green that make these sentences true for you.

1. I am   used to / not used to   speaking English with native speakers.

2. I am   accustomed to / not accustomed to   speaking English without translating from my language.

3. I am   getting used to / not getting used to   English slang.

4. I am   getting accustomed to / not getting accustomed to   reading English without using a dictionary.

## 10-10 Using *Be Used/Accustomed To* and *Get Used/Accustomed To*

| | |
|---|---|
| (a) I *am used to* hot weather.<br><br>(b) I *am accustomed to* hot weather.<br><br>(c) I *am used to living* in a hot climate.<br><br>(d) I *am accustomed to living* in a hot climate. | Examples (a) and (b) have the same meaning: "Living in a hot climate is usual and normal for me. I'm familiar with what it is like to live in a hot climate. Hot weather isn't strange or different to me."<br><br>Note in (c) and (d): *to* (a preposition) is followed by the *-ing* form of a verb (a gerund). |
| (e) I just moved from Florida to Alaska. I *am getting used to* (*accustomed to*) the cold weather here. | *get used to* / *accustomed to* = *become used to* |

### EXERCISE 49 ▶ Looking at grammar. (Chart 10-10)
**Part I.** Complete the sentences with *be used to,* affirmative or negative.

1. Juan is from Mexico. He _____is used to_____ hot weather. He _____isn't used to_____ cold weather.

2. Alice was born and raised in Miami. She _____ living in a big city.

3. My hometown is Dallas, but this year I'm moving to a small town. I _____

   living in a small town. I _____ living in a big city.

**Part II.** Complete the sentences with *be accustomed to,* affirmative or negative.

4. Spiro recently moved to Hong Kong from Greece. He _____is accustomed to_____ eating Greek

   food. He _____isn't accustomed to_____ eating Chinese food.

5. I always get up around 6:00 A.M. I _____ getting up early.

   I _____ sleeping late.

6. Our teacher always gives us a lot of homework. We _____ having

   a lot of homework every day.

### EXERCISE 50 ▶ Let's talk: interview. (Chart 10-10)
Ask questions with *be used to*/*accustomed to*. Share some answers with the class.

*Example:* buy \ frozen food
   → *Are you used to / accustomed to buying frozen food?*

| | | |
|---|---|---|
| 1. get up \ early | 4. skip \ lunch | 7. have \ dessert at night |
| 2. sleep \ late | 5. eat \ a late dinner | 8. live \ in a big city |
| 3. eat \ breakfast | 6. drink \ coffee in the morning | 9. pay \ for all your expenses |

### EXERCISE 51 ▶ Let's talk. (Chart 10-10)
Work in small groups. Answer the questions.

1. Think of a time you traveled to another country. What did you need to get used to?
2. Think about English. What have you gotten used to or not gotten used to?
3. Think about different stages of life. What do people need to get accustomed to as they age?

**EXERCISE 52 ▶ Reading and grammar.** (Charts 10-1 → 10-10)

**Part I.** Read the blog by co-author Stacy Hagen. <u>Underline</u> five examples of sentences with the grammar you have studied in this chapter. Refer to the charts if necessary.

# BlackBookBlog

## Cultural Differences

As you know, every country has different customs, and it can take a while to get used to them. I'd like to tell you about some customs on the West Coast of the United States, where I live. Most are pretty typical for the rest of the country, too.

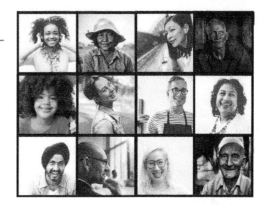

Although it is becoming more common to take shoes off, many people are still used to wearing them in the house. Sometimes people have a sign near the front door that says, "Please remove your shoes." Or you may be asked by your host to take them off. If you are not sure what to do, you can always ask your host. When I visit someone, I always take off my shoes and leave them near the door because I am used to doing this at my home.

When people are out walking and see someone they know, they like to smile and say, "Hi, how are you?" But this is just a quick greeting. They don't expect the other person to give a long answer. A common response is, "Pretty good, how are you?" Even when people aren't feeling so good, they often respond in a positive way. It may seem a little false, but it's just a greeting, not the start of a long conversation.

At school, teachers don't like to be interrupted in class. If a student is late, he or she enters quietly and sits at the side or the back of the room, if possible. Knocking is not necessary, and the noise bothers some teachers.

Generally, *Mr., Mrs.*, or *Ms.* is used with a teacher's last name in grades K–12. *Teacher* by itself is never used. In colleges and universities, the rules become a little more complicated. Some professors want you to use their first names. They will probably tell you this. But many are accustomed to the more formal *Professor* or *Doctor*. Sometimes your instructors will be teaching assistants who are students in graduate school. Often, first names are used, but some may ask that you use *Mr.* or *Ms. Professor* or *Doctor* is not appropriate with teaching assistants because they are not finished with their studies. If you are not sure, ask at the beginning of the term.

When people go to restaurants, it is common to leave tips for restaurant meals. Generally, the tip is left on the table or added to the credit card receipt. A tip of 15% is average. Some people tip 20–25% for excellent service. Some people will leave 10%, or even no tip, if they are not happy with the service. Money is not generally handed to the server.

It is good to research customs like these before you go to study or live in another country. Learning a language is hard, and you will feel more comfortable if you are acquainted with cultural differences.

**Part II.** Choose the answers for the customs in your country. Discuss them in groups and share a few of the answers with the class.

1. When I go to someone's home, shoes _____.
   a. are left outside the door
   b. are taken off after entering
   c. are kept on

2. When I am late for class, I _____.
   a. walk in and tell the teacher I am sorry
   b. walk in quietly and sit in the back of the room
   c. knock on the door and wait for the teacher to answer
   d. knock on the door one time and walk in

3. When I say my teacher's name, I use _____.
   a. the title (*Professor, Dr., Ms., Mr.*) and last name
   b. the first name only
   c. *Teacher* with no name
   d. *Sir, Madam,* or *Ma'am* with no name

4. After a meal at a restaurant, a tip _____.
   a. isn't left
   b. is left on the table
   c. is put on a credit card
   d. is handed to the server

**EXERCISE 53 ▶ Warm-up.** (Chart 10-11)
Complete the sentences about food preferences. Make statements that are true for you.

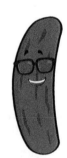

1. There are some foods I liked when I was younger, but now I don't eat them.

   I used to eat _____, but now I don't.

2. There are some foods I didn't like when I first tried them, but now they're OK.

   For example, the first time I ate _____, I didn't like

   it/them, but now I'm used to eating it/them.

| **10-11**  *Used To* vs. *Be Used To* | |
|---|---|
| (a) I *used to live* in Chicago, but now I live in Tokyo.<br>INCORRECT: *I used to living in Chicago.* | In (a): **Used to** expresses the habitual past (see Chart 2-9, p. 60). It is followed by the *simple form of a verb*. |
| (b) I *am used to living* in a big city.<br>INCORRECT: *I am used to live in a big city.* | In (b): **be used to** is followed by the **-ing** *form of a verb* (a gerund).* |

*NOTE: In both **used to** (habitual past) and **be used to**, the "d" is not pronounced in casual speech.

## EXERCISE 54 ▶ Looking at grammar. (Chart 10-11)

Complete the sentences with an appropriate form of **be**. If no form of **be** is necessary, use **Ø**.

1. a. I have lived in Malaysia for a long time.  I ___am___ used to warm weather.

   b. I ___Ø___ used to live in Portugal, but now I live in Spain.

2. a. I _____ used to sit in the back of the classroom, but now I prefer to sit in the front row.

   b. I _____ used to sitting at this desk.  I sit here every day.

3. a. When I was a child, I _____ used to play games with my friends in a big field near my house after school every day.

   b. It's hard for my kids to stay inside on a cold, rainy day.  They _____ used to playing outside in the big field near our house.  They play there almost every day.

4. a. A teacher _____ used to answering questions.  Students, especially good students, always have a lot of questions.

   b. I _____ used to be afraid to ask questions, but now I'm not.

5. a. People _____ used to believe the world was flat.

   b. I _____ used to believe that people on TV could see me.

## EXERCISE 55 ▶ Looking at grammar. (Chart 10-11)

Complete the sentences with **used to/be used to** and the correct form of the verb in parentheses.

Habits

1. Nick stays up later now than he did when he was in high school.  He (go) ___used to go___ to bed at ten, but now he rarely gets to bed before midnight.

2. I got used to going to bed late when I was in college, but now I have a job and I need my sleep.
   These days I (go) ___am used to going___ to bed around ten-thirty.

3. I am a vegetarian.  I (eat) _____ meat, but now I eat only meatless meals.

4. Ms. Wu has had a vegetable garden all her life.  She (grow) _____ her own vegetables.

5. Oscar has lived in Brazil for ten years.  He (eat) _____ Brazilian food.  It's his favorite.

6. Georgio moved to Germany to open his own restaurant.  He (have) _____
   _____ a small bakery in Italy.

7. I have taken the bus to work every day for the past five years.  I (take) _____
   _____ the bus.

8. Juanita travels by train on company business.  She (go) _____
   by plane, but now it's too expensive.

**EXERCISE 56 ▶ Warm-up.** (Chart 10-12)

Complete the sentences about airline passengers.

1. Before getting on the plane, passengers are expected to ...

2. After boarding the plane, passengers are supposed to ...

3. During landing, passengers are not supposed to ...

| 10-12 | Using *Be Supposed To* | |
|---|---|---|
| (a) | Mike *is supposed to call* me tomorrow.<br>(IDEA: I expect Mike to call me tomorrow.) | *Be supposed to* is used to talk about an activity or event that is expected to occur. |
| (b) | We *are supposed to write* a composition.<br>(IDEA: The teacher expects us to write a composition.) | In (a): The idea of *is supposed to* is that Mike is expected (by me) to call me. I asked him to call me. He promised to call me. I expect him to call me. |
| (c) | Alice *was supposed to be* home at ten, but she didn't get in until midnight.<br>(IDEA: Someone expected Alice to be home at ten.) | In the past form, *be supposed to* often expresses the idea that an expected event did not occur, as in (c). |

**EXERCISE 57 ▶ Looking at grammar.** (Chart 10-12)

Use *be supposed to*. Make a sentence with a similar meaning.

1. The teacher expects us to be on time for class.
   → *We are supposed to be on time for class.*
2. People expect the weather to be cold tomorrow.
3. People expect the plane to arrive at 6:00.
4. My boss expects me to work late tonight.
5. I expected the mail to come an hour ago, but it didn't.

**EXERCISE 58 ▶ Let's talk.** (Chart 10-12)

Read the list of stereotypes. Stereotypes are beliefs that many people may have. Work with a partner. Which ones do you agree with? Which ones do you disagree with? Explain your answers.

Stereotypes

1. Little girls are supposed to play with dolls.
2. Little boys are supposed to play with toy soldiers.
3. Women are supposed to be the main caregiver for the children.
4. Women are not supposed to have careers outside the home.
5. Men are not supposed to spend much time doing housework.
6. Men are supposed to be tough.
7. Women are not supposed to fight in wars.
8. Men are supposed to act strong.
9. Women are supposed to please people.

**EXERCISE 59 ▸ Check your knowledge.** (Chapter 10 Review)

Correct the errors.

1. I am agree with him.

2. Something was happened.

3. This pen is belong to me.

4. I'm interesting in that subject.

5. He is marry with my cousin.

6. Mary's dog was died last week.

7. Were you surprise when you heard the news?

8. When I went downtown, I am get lost.

9. The bus was arrived ten minutes late.

10. We're not suppose to have pets in our apartment.

**EXERCISE 60 ▸ Reading and writing.** (Chapter 10)

**Part I.** Read the passage and <u>underline</u> the passive verbs.

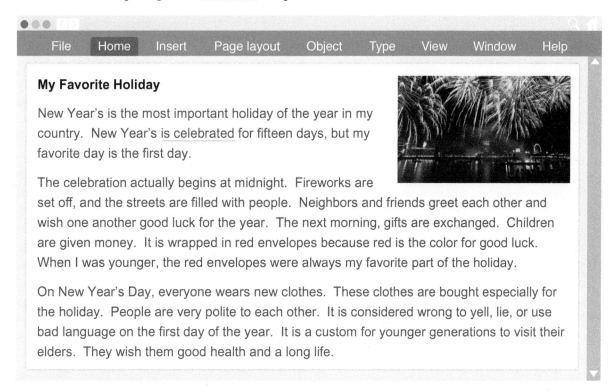

**My Favorite Holiday**

New Year's is the most important holiday of the year in my country. New Year's is celebrated for fifteen days, but my favorite day is the first day.

The celebration actually begins at midnight. Fireworks are set off, and the streets are filled with people. Neighbors and friends greet each other and wish one another good luck for the year. The next morning, gifts are exchanged. Children are given money. It is wrapped in red envelopes because red is the color for good luck. When I was younger, the red envelopes were always my favorite part of the holiday.

On New Year's Day, everyone wears new clothes. These clothes are bought especially for the holiday. People are very polite to each other. It is considered wrong to yell, lie, or use bad language on the first day of the year. It is a custom for younger generations to visit their elders. They wish them good health and a long life.

**Part II.** Choose a holiday you like. Describe the activities on this day. What do you do in the morning? Afternoon? Evening? Which activities do you enjoy the most? Make some of your sentences passive, as appropriate.

---

**WRITING TIP**

In most cases, it is better to use active verbs in writing. However, the passive is used when the doer of the action is not important or does not need to be mentioned. Here are some examples from the reading:

Fireworks are set off.          (not necessary to say: People set off fireworks.)
Money is given to children.     (not necessary to say: People give money to children.)
These clothes are bought        (not necessary to say: People buy clothes especially
especially for the holiday.     for the holiday.)

In each of these examples, use of the passive allows the reader to focus on what is most important, the receiver of the action: the fireworks, money, and the clothes.

---

**Part III.** Edit your writing. Check for the following:

1. ☐ a form of **be** for every passive verb
2. ☐ a past participle for every passive verb
3. ☐ use of the passive when the doer of the action does not need to be mentioned
4. ☐ a description of the day's activities
5. ☐ correct spelling (use a dictionary or spell-check)

---

▪▪▪▪▪ For digital resources, go to the Pearson Practice English app.

# CHAPTER 11

## Count/Noncount Nouns and Articles

---

**PRETEST: What do I already know?**

Write "C" if the **boldfaced** words are correct and "I" if they are incorrect.

1. _____ I live in **a** old house.  (Chart 11-1)

2. _____ We have **new furniture**.  (Chart 11-2)

3. _____ Would you like **a** rice?  (Chart 11-3)

4. _____ Many cities have **pollution**.  (Chart 11-4)

5. _____ I need to buy **a** some toothpaste.  I'm almost out.  (Chart 11-5)

6. _____ Do you take **a little** sugar in your coffee?  (Chart 11-5)

7. _____ My mom can't read small print any longer.  She needs to buy **glasses**.
   (Chart 11-6)

8. _____ Did you pick up **carton** of eggs at the store?  (Chart 11-7)

9. _____ My favorite foods are **apples** and chocolate.  (Chart 11-8)

10. _____ This is **the** second time that Mr. Reyes has asked for help.  (Chart 11-9)

11. _____ The tallest mountains in South America are **the** Andes.  (Chart 11-10)

12. _____ Tina likes to walk in **Central Park** for exercise.  (Chart 11-11)

---

**EXERCISE 1 ▸ Warm-up.**  (Chart 11-1)

Check (✓) all the items you have with you right now.  Do you know why some nouns have **a** before them and others have **an?**

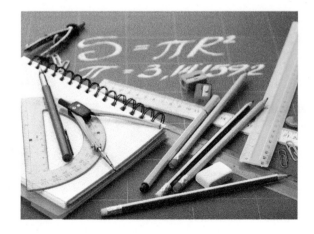

1. _____ **a** ruler

2. _____ **an** eraser

3. _____ **a** paper clip

4. _____ **an** umbrella

5. _____ **a** used textbook

6. _____ **a** university map

## 11-1 A vs. An

| | |
|---|---|
| (a) I have *a pencil*.<br>(b) I live in *an apartment*.<br>(c) I have *a small apartment*.<br>(d) I live in *an old building*. | *A* and *an* are used in front of a singular noun (e.g., *pencil, apartment*). They mean "one."<br><br>If a singular noun is modified by an adjective (e.g., *small, old*), *a* or *an* comes in front of the adjective, as in (c) and (d).<br><br>*A* is used in front of words that begin with a consonant (*b, c, d, f, g,* etc.): *a boy, a bad day, a cat, a cute baby*.<br><br>*An* is used in front of words that begin with the vowels *a*, *e*, *i*, and *o*: *an apartment, an angry man, an elephant, an empty room*, etc. |
| (e) I have *an umbrella*.<br>(f) I saw *an ugly picture*.<br>(g) I attend *a university*.<br>(h) I had *a unique experience*. | For words that begin with the letter *u*:<br>   (1) *An* is used if the *u* is a vowel sound, as in *an umbrella, an uncle, an unusual day*.<br>   (2) *A* is used if the *u* is a consonant sound, as in *a university, a unit, a usual event*. |
| (i) He will arrive in *an hour*.<br>(j) New Year's Day is *a holiday*. | For words that begin with the letter *h*:<br>   (1) *An* is used if the *h* is silent: *an hour, an honor, an honest person*.<br>   (2) *A* is used if the *h* is pronounced: *a holiday, a hotel, a high grade*. |

### EXERCISE 2 ▸ Looking at grammar. (Chart 11-1)
Add *a* or *an* to these words.

1. __a__ mistake
2. _____ abbreviation
3. _____ dream
4. _____ interesting dream
5. _____ empty box
6. _____ box
7. _____ uniform
8. _____ email
9. _____ untrue story
10. _____ unusual message
11. _____ universal problem
12. _____ unhappy child
13. _____ hour or two
14. _____ hole in the ground
15. _____ hill
16. _____ handsome man
17. _____ honest man
18. _____ honor

### EXERCISE 3 ▸ Grammar and speaking. (Chart 11-1)
Add *a* or *an*. Take turns telling your partner what you did and didn't eat last week.

***Example:*** I had an egg. I didn't have a banana. Etc.

1. _____ egg
2. _____ banana
3. _____ orange
4. _____ carrot
5. _____ tomato
6. _____ sandwich
7. _____ bowl of ice cream
8. _____ apple
9. _____ potato
10. _____ salty snack
11. _____ icy drink
12. _____ healthy meal

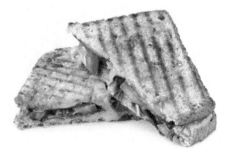

## EXERCISE 4 ▶ Warm-up. (Chart 11-2)
Choose the correct completions. More than one answer may be correct.

1. I need one _____.
   a. chair            b. chairs

2. There are two _____ in the room.
   a. chairs           b. furniture

3. I found some _____ in the storage room.
   a. chair            b. furniture

4. I found _____ in the storage room.
   a. chairs           b. furniture

| 11-2 | Count and Noncount Nouns | | |
|---|---|---|---|
| | **Singular** | **Plural** | |
| COUNT NOUN | *a* chair <br> *one* chair | Ø chairs <br> *two* chairs <br> *some* chairs | A count noun: <br> (1) can be counted with numbers: *one chair, two chairs, ten chairs, etc.* <br> (2) can be preceded by *a/an* in the singular: *a chair.* <br> (3) has a plural form ending in *-s* or *-es: chairs.** |
| NONCOUNT NOUN | Ø furniture <br> *some* furniture | Ø <br> Ø | A noncount noun: <br> (1) cannot be counted with numbers. <br>    INCORRECT: *one furniture* <br> (2) is NOT immediately preceded by *a/an*. <br>    INCORRECT: *a furniture* <br> (3) does NOT have a plural form (no final *-s*). <br>    INCORRECT: *furnitures* |

*See Chart 1-4, p. 11, Chart 6-1, p. 158, and Appendix A-6 for the spelling and pronunciation of *-s/-es*.

## EXERCISE 5 ▶ Looking at grammar. (Chart 11-2)
Check (✓) the correct sentences. Correct the sentences with errors. Use ***some*** with the noncount nouns.

1. __✓__ I bought one chair for my apartment.
2. _____ I bought one furniture for my apartment.* *(some)*
3. _____ I bought four chairs for my apartment.
4. _____ I bought four furnitures for my apartment.
5. _____ I bought a chair for my apartment.
6. _____ I bought a furniture for my apartment.
7. _____ I bought some chair for my apartment.
8. _____ I bought some furnitures for my apartment.

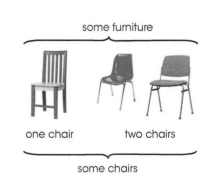

some furniture

one chair     two chairs

some chairs

---

*CORRECT: *I bought **some furniture** for my apartment.* OR *I bought **furniture** for my apartment.* See Chart 11–5 for more information about the use of **Ø** and ***some***.

## EXERCISE 6 ▸ Warm-up. (Chart 11-3)

Write the words in the correct columns.

| bills | ideas | necklaces | rings | tips |
|-------|-------|-----------|-------|------|
| bracelets | letters | postcards | suggestions | |

| ADVICE | MAIL | JEWELRY |
|--------|------|---------|
| _____ | _____ | _____ |
| _____ | _____ | _____ |
| _____ | _____ | _____ |

## 11-3 Noncount Nouns

| | |
|---|---|
| **Individual Parts → The Whole**<br>(Count Nouns)　(Noncount Nouns)<br><br>(a) letters<br>　　postcards<br>　　bills　→ *mail*<br>　　etc.<br><br>(b) apples<br>　　bananas<br>　　oranges　→ *fruit*<br>　　etc.<br><br>(c) rings<br>　　bracelets<br>　　necklaces　→ *jewelry*<br>　　etc. | Noncount nouns usually refer to a whole group of things that is made up of many individual parts, a whole category made of different varieties.<br><br>For example, *furniture* is a noncount noun; it describes a whole category of things: *chairs, tables, beds, etc.*<br><br>　　chairs<br>　　tables<br>　　beds　→ **furniture**<br>　　etc.<br><br>*Mail, fruit,* and *jewelry* are other examples of noncount nouns that refer to a whole category made up of individual parts. |

### Some Common Noncount Nouns: Whole Groups Made up of Individual Parts

| A. | B. | E. | G. |
|----|----|----|----|
| baggage | homework | grammar | chalk |
| clothing | housework | slang | corn |
| equipment | work | vocabulary | dirt |
| food | | | flour |
| furniture | C. advice | F. Arabic | hair |
| luggage | information | Chinese | pepper |
| money | | English | rice |
| scenery | D. history | German | salt |
| stuff | literature | Indonesian | sand |
| traffic | music | Spanish | sugar |
| | poetry | | |

**EXERCISE 7 ▶ Looking at grammar.** (Charts 11-2 and 11-3)

Complete the sentences with *a*/*an* or *some*. Decide if the nouns in green are count or noncount.

| | | | |
|---|---|---|---|
| 1. I often have _____*some*_____ fruit for dessert. | | count | (noncount) |
| 2. I had _____*a*_____ peach for dessert. | | (count) | noncount |
| 3. I got _____ letter today. | | count | noncount |
| 4. I got _____ mail today. | | count | noncount |
| 5. Anna wears _____ ring on her left hand. | | count | noncount |
| 6. Maria is wearing _____ jewelry today. | | count | noncount |
| 7. I have _____ homework to finish. | | count | noncount |
| 8. I have _____ assignment to finish. | | count | noncount |
| 9. I needed _____ information. | | count | noncount |
| 10. I asked _____ question. | | count | noncount |

**EXERCISE 8 ▶ Grammar and speaking.** (Charts 11-2 and 11-3)

Add final *-s*/*-es* if possible. Otherwise, write **Ø**. Then decide if you agree or disagree with the statement. Discuss your answers.

Opinions

| | | |
|---|---|---|
| 1. I'm learning a lot of **grammar**__*Ø*__ this term. | yes | no |
| 2. Count and noncount **noun**_*s*_ are easy. | yes | no |
| 3. A good way to control **traffic**_____ is to charge people money to drive in the city. | yes | no |
| 4. Electric **car**_____ will replace gas **car**_____. | yes | no |
| 5. **Information**_____ from the internet is usually reliable. | yes | no |
| 6. **Fact**_____ are always true. | yes | no |
| 7. Many **word**_____ in English are similar to those in my language. | yes | no |
| 8. The best way to learn new **vocabulary**_____ is to memorize it. | yes | no |
| 9. I enjoy singing karaoke **song**_____. | yes | no |
| 10. I enjoy listening to classical **music**_____. | yes | no |
| 11. I like to read good **literature**_____. | yes | no |
| 12. I like to read mystery **novel**_____. | yes | no |
| 13. **Beach**_____ are relaxing places to visit. | yes | no |
| 14. Walking on **sand**_____ is good exercise for your legs. | yes | no |
| 15. Parents usually have helpful **suggestion**_____ for their kids. | yes | no |
| 16. Sometimes kids have helpful **advice**_____ for their parents. | yes | no |

## EXERCISE 9 ▸ Warm-up. (Chart 11-4)

Complete the sentences with words in the box. Make sentences that are true for you.

| | | | | |
|---|---|---|---|---|
| beauty | health | milk | pollution | traffic |
| coffee | honesty | money | smog | violence |
| happiness | juice | noise | tea | water |

1. During the day, I drink _____ or _____ .

2. Two things I don't like about big cities are _____ and

   _____ .

3. _____ is more important than _____ .

## 11-4 More Noncount Nouns

| (a) **Liquids** | | **Solids and Semi-Solids** | | | | **Gases** |
|---|---|---|---|---|---|---|
| coffee | soup | bread | meat | glass | paper | air |
| milk | tea | butter | beef | silver | soap | pollution |
| oil | water | cheese | chicken | gold | toothpaste | smog |
| | | ice | fish | iron | wood | smoke |

| (b) **Things That Occur in Nature** | | | | | | |
|---|---|---|---|---|---|---|
| weather | darkness | sunshine | | | | |
| rain | light | thunder | | | | |
| snow | sunlight | lightning | | | | |

| (c) **Abstractions*** | | | | | | |
|---|---|---|---|---|---|---|
| beauty | fun | health | ignorance | love | peace | time |
| courage | generosity | help | kindness | luck | progress | violence |
| experience | happiness | honesty | knowledge | patience | selfishness | |

*An abstraction is an idea. It has no physical form. A person cannot touch it.

## EXERCISE 10 ▸ Looking at grammar. (Charts 11-2 → 11-4)

Add final *-s*/*-es* if possible. Otherwise, write **Ø**. Choose the correct verb as necessary.

1. I made some **mistake** _s___ on my algebra test.

2. In the winter in Siberia, there (is) / are **snow** _Ø___ on the ground.

3. Siberia has very cold **weather** _____ .

4. Be sure to give the new couple my best **wish** _____ .

5. I want to wish them good **luck** _____ .

6. **Silver** _____ is / are expensive. **Diamond** _____ is / are expensive too.

7. I admire Professor Yoo for her extensive **knowledge** _____ of organic farming methods.

8. Professor Yoo has a lot of good **idea** _____ and strong **opinion** _____ .

9. Teaching children to read requires **patience**_____.

10. Doctors take care of **patient**_____.

11. Mr. Fernandez's English is improving. He's making **progress**_____.

12. Wood stoves are a source of **pollution** _____ in many cities.

## EXERCISE 11 ▸ Listening. (Charts 11-2 → 11-4)
Listen to the sentences. Add **-s** if the given nouns have plural endings. Otherwise, write **Ø**.

*Example:* You will hear: Watch out! The steps are icy.

You will write: step _s_____

1. chalk_____                6. storm_____

2. soap_____                 7. storm_____

3. suggestion_____           8. toothpaste_____

4. suggestion_____           9. stuff_____

5. gold_____                 10. equipment_____

## EXERCISE 12 ▸ Let's talk. (Chart 11-4)
Work in small groups. Can you figure out the meaning of each saying? Choose one to explain to the class.

Common Sayings

*Example:* Ignorance is bliss.

→ **Ignorance** *means you don't know about something.* **Bliss** *means "happiness."*
*This saying means that you are happier if you don't know about a problem.*

1. Honesty is the best policy.
2. Time is money.
3. Laughter is the best medicine.
4. Knowledge is power.
5. Experience is the best teacher.

## EXERCISE 13 ▸ Let's talk. (Chart 11-4)
Complete the sentences. Give two to four answers for each item. Share your answers with a partner. See how many of your answers are the same. REMINDER: Abstract nouns are usually noncount. To find out if a noun is count or noncount, check your dictionary or ask your teacher.

*In my opinion ...*

1. some nice qualities in a person are ...
2. some bad qualities people can have are ...
3. some of the most important things in life are ...
4. certain bad conditions exist in the world. Some of them are ...
5. some things in nature that cause problems are ...

**EXERCISE 14 ▶ Game.** (Charts 11-1 → 11-4)

Work in small teams. Imagine your team is at one of the places in the box. Make a list of the things you see. Share your team's list with the class. The team with the most complete and grammatically correct list wins.

| | | |
|---|---|---|
| a restaurant | an island | an airport |
| a museum | a hotel | a popular department store |

*Example:* a teacher's office

→ *two windows*
→ *a lot of grammar books*
→ *office equipment — a computer, a printer*
→ *office supplies — a stapler, paper clips, pens, pencils, a ruler*
→ *some pictures*
→ *some furniture*
→ *three chairs*
→ *a backpack*
→ *two bookshelves*
   *etc.*

**EXERCISE 15 ▶ Warm-up.** (Chart 11-5)

Complete the sentences with **apples** or **fruit**.

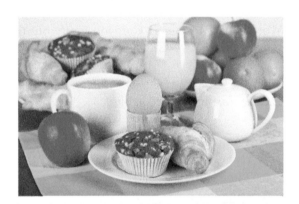

1. I bought several _____ yesterday.

2. Do you eat a lot of _____?

3. Do you eat many _____?

4. Do you eat much _____?

5. I eat a few _____ every week.

6. I eat a little _____ for breakfast.

## 11-5 Using *A Lot Of, Some, Several, Many/Much,* and *A Few/A Little*

| | Count | Noncount | |
|---|---|---|---|
| (a) | *a lot of* chairs | *a lot of* furniture | **A lot of** and **some** are used with both count and noncount nouns. |
| (b) | *some* chairs | *some* furniture | |
| (c) | *several* chairs | Ø | **Several** is used only with count nouns. |
| (d) | *many* chairs | *much* furniture | **Many** is used with count nouns.<br>**Much** is used with noncount nouns. |
| (e) | *a few* chairs | *a little* furniture | **A few** is used with count nouns.<br>**A little** is used with noncount nouns. |

## EXERCISE 16 ▸ Looking at grammar. (Charts 11-2 and 11-5)

Check (✓) the correct sentences. Correct the sentences that have errors. One sentence has a spelling error.

1. _____ Jakob learned s̶e̶v̶e̶r̶a̶l̶ *some/Ø* new vocabulary.

2. _✓_ He learned several new words.

3. _____ Takashi learned a lot of new words.

4. _____ Sonia learned a lot of new vocabulary too.

5. _____ Lydia doesn't like learning too much new vocabulary in one day.

6. _____ She can't remember too much new words.

7. _____ Mr. Lee assigned a few vocabulary to his class.

8. _____ He assigned a few new words.

9. _____ He explained several new vocabulary.

10. _____ There is alot of new word at this level.

11. _____ There are a lot of new vocabulary at this level.

## EXERCISE 17 ▸ Looking at grammar: pairwork. (Charts 11-2 → 11-5)

Work with a partner. Take turns completing the questions with **How many** or **How much** and each of the given nouns.* Make the nouns plural as necessary.

1. How _____ does Mr. Miller have?
   a. son → *many sons*
   b. child → *many children*
   c. work → *much work*
   d. car
   e. stuff
   f. experience

2. How _____ did you buy?
   a. fruit
   b. vegetable
   c. banana
   d. tomato
   e. orange
   f. food

3. How _____ did you have?
   a. fun
   b. help
   c. time
   d. information
   e. fact
   f. money

---

*****Much** and **many** are more commonly used in questions than in affirmative statements.

## EXERCISE 18 ▸ Let's talk: interview. (Chart 11-5)

Interview your classmates. Begin your questions with **How much** or **How many**. Share some of your answers with the class.

*How much/How many ...*

1. pages does this book have?
2. coffee do you drink every day?
3. cups of tea do you drink every day?
4. homework do you have to do tonight?
5. assignments have you had this week?
6. many times during the week do you make your own lunch?
7. many hours do you usually sleep at night?
8. snow does this area get in the winter?

## EXERCISE 19 ▸ Looking at grammar. (Charts 11-2 → 11-5)

Complete the sentences with **a few** or **a little** and the given noun. Use the plural form of the noun as necessary.

1. *music*     I feel like listening to _____*a little music*_____ tonight.

2. *song*     We sang _____*a few songs*_____ at the party.

3. *help*     Do you need _____ with that?

4. *pepper*     The soup just needs _____.

5. *thing*     I need to pick up _____ at the store on my way home from work tonight.

6. *apple*     I bought _____ at the store.*

7. *fruit*     I bought _____ at the store.

8. *advice*     I need _____.

9. *money*     If I accept that job, I'll make _____ more _____.

10. *friend*     _____ came by last night to visit us.

11. *rain*     It looks like we might get _____ today. I think I'll take my umbrella with me.

12. *French*     I can speak _____, but I don't know any Italian at all.

13. *hour*     Ron's plane will arrive in _____ more _____.

---

*\*I bought a few apples.* = I bought a small number of apples.
*I bought a little apple.* = I bought one apple, and it was small, not large.

## EXERCISE 20 ▶ Warm-up. (Chart 11-6)

Match the sentences to the pictures.

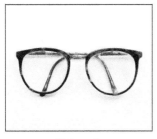

Picture A

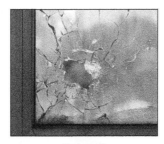

Picture B

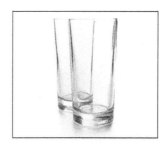

Picture C

1. Do you need one glass or two? _____

2. Your glasses fit nicely. _____

3. A: What happened?

   B: Some kids threw a ball and hit the glass. _____

## 11-6 Nouns That Can Be Count or Noncount

Quite a few nouns can be used as either count or noncount nouns. Examples of both count and noncount usages for some common nouns follow.

| Noun | Used as a Noncount Noun | Used as a Count Noun |
|------|-------------------------|----------------------|
| glass | (a) Windows are made of *glass*. | (b) I drank *a glass* of water. |
|       |                                  | (c) Janet wears *glasses* when she reads. |
| hair | (d) Rita has brown *hair*. | (e) There's *a hair* on my jacket. |
| iron | (f) *Iron* is a metal. | (g) I pressed my shirt with *an iron*. |
| light | (h) I opened the curtain to let in *some light*. | (i) Please turn off *the lights* (lamps). |
| paper | (j) I need *some paper* to write a note. | (k) I wrote *a paper* for Professor Lee. |
|       |                                                 | (l) I bought *a paper* (a newspaper). |
| time | (m) How *much time* do you need to finish your work? | (n) How *many times* have you been to Mexico? |
| work | (o) I have *some work* to do tonight. | (p) That painting is *a work* of art. |
| coffee | (q) I had *some coffee* after dinner. | (r) *Two coffees*, please. |
| chicken/fish | (s) I ate *some chicken/some fish*. | (t) She drew a picture of *a chicken/a fish*. |
| experience | (u) I haven't had *much experience* with this software. (I don't have much knowledge or skill with this software.) | (v) I had *many* interesting *experiences* on my trip. (Many interesting events happened to me on my trip.) |

## EXERCISE 21 ▸ Looking at grammar. (Chart 11-6)
Match the correct picture to each sentence. Discuss the differences in meaning.

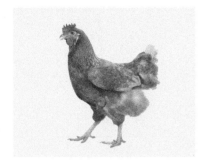
Picture A

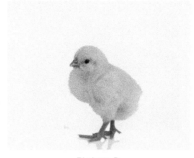
Picture B

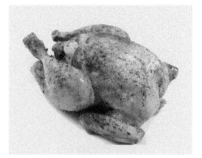
Picture C

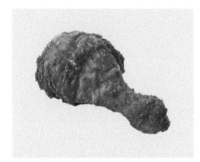
Picture D

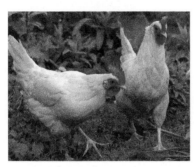
Picture E

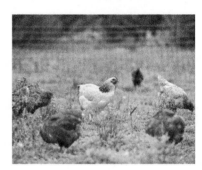
Picture F

1. That was a great meal. I ate a lot of chicken. Now I'm stuffed.* _____

2. Are you hungry? How about a little chicken for lunch? _____

3. When I was a child, we raised several chickens. _____

4. I bought a couple of chickens so I can have fresh eggs. _____

5. There's a little chicken in your yard. _____

6. That's a big chicken over there. Who does it belong to? _____

## EXERCISE 22 ▸ Looking at grammar. (Chart 11-6)
Complete the sentences with the given words. Make words plural as necessary. Choose words in green as necessary. Discuss the differences in meaning.

1. *time*
   a. It took a lot of ___*time*___ to write my composition.
   b. I really like that movie. I saw it three ___*times*___.

2. *paper*
   a. Students in Professor Young's literature class have to write a lot of _____.
   b. Students who take careful lecture notes can use a lot of _____.
   c. The *New York Times* is   a / some   famous _____.

---

*\*stuffed* = very full

3. *work*

   a. Van Gogh's painting *Irises* is a beautiful _____ of art.

   b. I have a lot of _____ to do tomorrow at my office.

4. *hair*

   a. Erin has straight _____, and Mariam has curly _____.

   b. Brian has a white cat. When I stood up from Brian's sofa, my black slacks were covered with short white _____.

5. *glass*

   a. I wear _____ for reading.

   b. In some countries, people use _____ for their tea; in other countries, they use cups.

   c. Many famous paintings are covered with _____ to protect them.

6. *iron*

   a. _____   is / are   necessary to animal and plant life.

   b. _____   is / are   used to make clothes look neat.

7. *experience*

   a. My grandfather had a lot of interesting _____ in his long career as a diplomat.

   b. You should apply for the job at the electronics company because you have a lot of _____ in that field.

8. *chicken*

   a. Joe, would you like   a / some   more _____?

   b. My grandmother raises _____ in her yard.

9. *light*

   a. There   is / are   a lot of _____ on the ceilings of the school building.

   b. A: If you want to take a picture outside now, you'll need a flash.  The _____ isn't / aren't   good here.

      B: Or, we could wait an hour.   It / They   will be brighter then.

## EXERCISE 23 ▶ Warm-up.  (Chart 11-7)
Which of the following do you have in your cupboard?  Check (✓) the items.

1. _____ a can* of tuna
2. _____ a bag of flour
3. _____ a jar of jam
4. _____ a bottle of soda pop
5. _____ a box of pasta
6. _____ a bowl of sugar

*a can* in American English = *a tin* in British English

## 11-7 Using Units of Measure with Noncount Nouns

| | |
|---|---|
| (a) I had some tea.<br>(b) I had *two cups of* tea. | To mention a specific quantity of a noncount noun, speakers use units of measure such as *two cups of* or *one piece of*. |
| (c) I ate some toast.<br>(d) I ate *one piece of* toast. | A unit of measure usually describes **the container** (*a cup of, a bowl of*), **the amount** (*a pound of, a quart of*),* or **the shape** (*a bar of soap, a sheet of paper*). |

*Weight measure: *one pound* = 0.45 kilograms/kilos.
 Liquid measure: *one quart* = 0.95 litres/liters; four quarts = one gallon = 3.8 litres/liters.

### EXERCISE 24 ▸ Let's talk. (Chart 11-7)

Work with a partner. Complete the conversation about lunchtime by combining the words in the box. Perform the conversation several times with different food choices. Take turns being Partner A and Partner B. You can look at your book before you speak. When you speak, look at your partner.

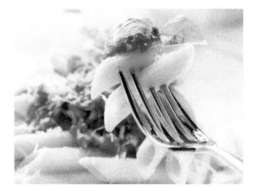

| | | |
|---|---|---|
| | bread | orange juice |
| a glass of | cake | pasta |
| a cup of | candy | pizza |
| a bowl of | cereal | popcorn |
| a slice of | cheese | rice |
| a piece of | chicken | soda |
| a dish of | ice cream | soup |
| a plate of | mineral water | strawberries |
| | noodles | watermelon |

*Example:*

PARTNER A: What are you having for lunch?
PARTNER B: I don't have much time. Maybe I'll just have _____.
PARTNER A: How about you?
PARTNER B: I'm really hungry. I think I'll have _____ and _____.

### EXERCISE 25 ▸ Looking at grammar. (Chart 11-7)

What units of measure are <u>usually</u> used with the given nouns? More than one unit of measure can be used with some of the nouns.

At the Store

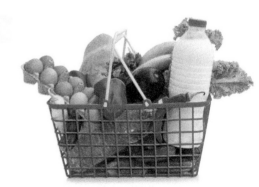

bag  bottle  box  can  carton  jar

1. a ____*can/jar*____ of olives
2. a ____*box/bag*____ of crackers
3. a _____ of mineral water
4. a _____ of jam or jelly

5. a _____ of tuna

6. a _____ of soup

7. a _____ of sugar

8. a _____ of milk

9. a _____ of soda

10. a _____ of flour

11. a _____ of pet food

12. a _____ of breakfast cereal

## EXERCISE 26 ▶ Let's talk. (Chart 11-7)

You and your partner are planning a party for the class. You still need to buy a few things at the store. Decide what you'd like to get using the sentences below as your guide. You can be serious or silly. Perform your conversation for the class. Then your classmates will tell you if they want to come to your party or not. NOTE: You can look at your conversation before you speak. When you speak, look at your partner.

**Shopping List**

A: So what else do we need from the store?

B: Let's see. We need a few jars of _____. We should also get a box of

_____. Oh, and a couple of bags of _____.

A: Is that it? Anything else?

B: I guess a few cans of _____ would be good. I almost forgot. What should

we do about drinks?

A: How about some bottles (or cans) of _____?

B: Good idea.

A: By the way, I thought we could serve slices of _____.

B: Sure.

## EXERCISE 27 ▶ Warm-up. (Chart 11-8)

Which sentence best describes each picture?

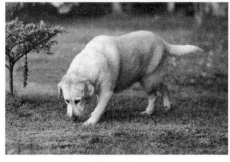

Picture A                    Picture B

1. I see a dog. _____

2. Do you know the dog in the yard? _____

3. I love dogs. _____

## 11-8 Articles with Count and Noncount Nouns: *A/an, The, Ø*

### Singular Count Nouns: *A/An* or *The*

| | |
|---|---|
|    <br><br>(a) Joe bought *a house*. | ***a/an*** = one<br>In (a): The speaker is not talking about a specific house. The speaker is talking about one house (of many).<br>A singular count noun must have an article.<br>*INCORRECT: Joe bought house.* |
| <br><br>(b) *The house* next door is for sale. | In (b): ***the*** = a specific house<br>*INCORRECT: House next door is for sale.* |

### Plural Count Nouns: *Ø* or *The*

| | |
|---|---|
|     <br><br>(c) *Ø Houses* are expensive. | In (c): ***Houses*** is non-specific, and no article is used. The speaker is talking about houses in general, not a specific group of houses.<br>***A*** is never used with plural count nouns.<br>*INCORRECT: A houses.*<br>See Chart 11-5 for other expressions that can be used such as ***some, several, a few, a lot of***. |
|   <br><br>(d) *The houses* in my neighborhood are very nice. | In (d): ***the*** = a specific group of houses, the houses in my neighborhood |

### Noncount Nouns: *Ø* or *The*

| | |
|---|---|
| 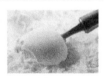<br><br>(e) I like *Ø ice cream*. | In (e): ***Ice cream*** is noncount. The speaker is talking about any ice cream, all ice cream, ice cream in general. |
| <br><br>(f) *The ice cream* in the dish is for you. | In (f): ***The*** is used because the speaker is talking about specific ice cream, the ice cream in the dish.<br>*INCORRECT: Ice cream in the dish is for you.* |

## EXERCISE 28 ▸ Looking at grammar. (Chart 11-8)

Decide if the words in green have a specific or non-specific meaning.

1. The keys on the counter are Jason's.          specific     non-specific
2. I saw a snake in the grass.          specific     non-specific

3. Do you like chocolate?                         specific    non-specific
4. The chocolate in the box is a gift.            specific    non-specific
5. I need information. Can you help me?           specific    non-specific
6. The information you gave me was helpful.       specific    non-specific

## EXERCISE 29 ▶ Looking at grammar. (Chart 11-8)
Write *a, the,* or *Ø*.

1. SPECIFIC: I need to repair _____ car.
   NON-SPECIFIC: I need to repair _____ car.

2. SPECIFIC: Do you have _____ homework?
   NON-SPECIFIC: Do you have _____ homework?

3. NON-SPECIFIC: _____ phone is ringing.
   SPECIFIC: _____ phone is ringing.

4. NON-SPECIFIC: A bag of flour is on _____ shelf.
   SPECIFIC: A bag of flour is on _____ shelf.

5. SPECIFIC: I love _____ tea.
   NON-SPECIFIC: I love _____ tea.

6. NON-SPECIFIC: I have _____ vegetables from our neighbor's garden.
   SPECIFIC: I have _____ vegetables from our neighbor's garden.

## EXERCISE 30 ▶ Looking at grammar. (Chart 11-8)
Read the conversations and decide whether the speakers would probably use *the* or *a*.

1. A: What did you do last night?
   B: I went to ____*a*____ party.
   A: Oh? Where was it?

2. A: Did you have a good time at ____*the*____ party last night?
   B: Yes.
   A: So did I. I'm glad that you decided to go with me.

3. A: Do you have _____ car?
   B: No. But I have _____ motorcycle.

4. A: Is Mr. Jones _____ graduate student?
   B: No. He's _____ professor.

5. A: I liked your presentation at _____ meeting yesterday.
   B: Thanks. I worked really hard on it.

6. A: Does San Diego have _____ zoo?
   B: Yes. It's world famous.

7. A: Did you like _____ apartment you saw yesterday?
   B: Yes. It has _____ big kitchen.

**EXERCISE 31** ▸ **Listening.** (Chart 11-8)

Articles are hard to hear. Listen to the conversation. Decide if you hear **a, an, the,** or **Ø** (no article).

**Example:** You will hear: I have an idea.
You will choose: a (an) the Ø

| | | | | | | | | |
|---|---|---|---|---|---|---|---|---|
| 1. a | an | the | Ø | | 6. a | an | the | Ø |
| 2. a | an | the | Ø | | 7. a | an | the | Ø |
| 3. a | an | the | Ø | | 8. a | an | the | Ø |
| 4. a | an | the | Ø | | 9. a | an | the | Ø |
| 5. a | an | the | Ø | | 10. a | an | the | Ø |

**EXERCISE 32** ▸ **Warm-up.** (Chart 11-9)

Look at the articles in green. Why do the speakers use **the?** Discuss your answers.

1. A: Did you find the keys?
   B: Not yet. I'm still looking for the light switch!
2. A: Where is the moon?
   B: It's behind the clouds.
3. A: Did you see Mika's pets?
   B: Yes, the dog is friendlier than the cat.

| 11-9 More About Articles | |
|---|---|
| (a) Did you feed *the dog*? <br> (b) Please turn off *the lights*. <br> (c) *The moon* is very bright tonight. <br> (d) Where is *the library*? | Use ***the*** when the speaker and listener are thinking about the same specific person or thing. <br><br> In (a): The speaker and the listener are thinking about the same dog, for example, the dog in their house. <br><br> In (b): The speaker and listener are thinking about the same lights, for example, the lights in the room. <br><br> In (c): There is only one moon for the speaker and listener to think of. <br><br> In (d): Both the speaker and listener know the library, for example, at their school, or in their town. |
| (e) I had *a banana* and ***an*** *apple*. I gave *the banana* to Joe. <br> (f) That was *a great meal*. *The food* was excellent. | Use ***the*** for the second mention of a noun, as in (e). The speaker and listener know whom or what is being talked about. <br><br> The noun in the second mention doesn't need to be the exact same word as in the first mention. In (f), ***food*** refers to ***meal***. |
| (g) I spoke with *Ø my advisor*. <br> (h) You need to take *Ø this bus*. <br> (i) Mari is *Ø helpful*. | Do not use articles before possessive adjectives (e.g., ***my***), demonstrative adjectives (e.g., ***this***), and adjectives by themselves. <br> INCORRECT: *a my advisor* <br>          *a this bus* <br>          *a helpful* |

| | |
|---|---|
| (j) What is *the first* step? <br> (k) *The last* time we met was in high school. <br> (l) This is *the second* time I've called. <br> (m) Tony and I have *the same* class schedule. <br> (n) What is *the best* solution? | In (j)–(l): Nouns with **first**, **last**, and ordinal numbers generally take **the**. <br><br> In (m) and (n): **Same** and **best** always takes **the**. |
| (o) Lyn is *in bed*. <br> (p) Andrew is *at school*. | Expressions that refer to activities do not use **the**. <br> In (o): Lyn is lying down, probably sleeping. <br> In (p): Andrew is studying. |

**Common Expressions Without *The***

in jail/prison (staying as a prisoner)
in class (studying)
in college (attending school—college or university)
at work  (working)
at church (praying)
at home (doing a variety of activities)

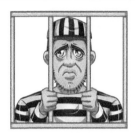

## EXERCISE 33 ▶ Looking at grammar. (Chart 11-9)
Complete the conversation with the correct articles.

Last-Minute Check

A: Did you lock _____ door?
    ¹

B: Yes.

A: Did you check _____ stove?
    ²

B: Yes.

A: Did you close all _____ windows downstairs?
    ³

B: Yes.

A: Did you set _____ alarm?
    ⁴

B: Yes.

A: Then let's turn out _____ lights.
    ⁵

B: Goodnight, dear.

A: Oh, don't forget your appointment

    with _____ doctor tomorrow.
    ⁶

B: Yes, dear. Goodnight.

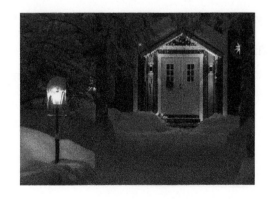

## EXERCISE 34 ▸ Looking at grammar. (Chart 11-9)
Choose the sentence that describes the given sentence.

1. We found the cat in the tree.
   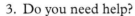
   a. We know the cat.
   b. We don't know the cat.

2. We found a cat in the tree.
   a. We know the cat.
   b. We don't know the cat.

3. Do you need help?
   a. Do you need specific help?
   b. Do you need help in general?

4. I left my car keys in the library.
   a. You know the library I am talking about.
   b. You don't know the library I am talking about.

5. Who fixed the TVs?
   a. I'm asking about TVs in general.
   b. I'm asking about specific TVs.

6. Mmmm. The coffee smells fresh.
   a. I'm talking about specific coffee.
   b. I'm talking about coffee in general.

## EXERCISE 35 ▸ Looking at grammar. (Chart 11-9)
Complete the sentences with *a/an* or *the*.

1. I had ___*a*___ banana and ___*an*___ apple. I gave ___*the*___ banana to Mary. I ate ___*the*___ apple.

2. I had _____ bananas and _____ apples. I gave _____ bananas to Mary. I ate _____ apples.

3. I forgot to bring my things with me to class yesterday, so I borrowed _____ pencil and _____ calculator from Joe. I returned _____ calculator, but I used _____ pencil for my homework.

4. A: What did you do last weekend?

   B: I went on _____ picnic Saturday and saw _____ movie Sunday.

   A: Did you have fun?

   B: _____ picnic was fun, but _____ movie was boring.

**EXERCISE 36 ▶ Looking at grammar.** (Chart 11-9)
Complete the sentences with *a, the,* or *Ø*.

**An Unlucky Purchase**

I bought _____ butter, eggs, and _____ bag
                 1                                    2

of flour to make _____ cookies. _____ butter and
                     3                       4

eggs were OK, but I had to return _____ flour. When I
                                      5

opened it, I found _____ little bugs in it. I took it back
                       6

to the people at the store and showed them _____ little bugs. They gave me _____ new bag
                                                7                                    8

of flour. _____ second bag didn't have any bugs in it.
             9

**EXERCISE 37 ▶ Looking at grammar.** (Charts 11-8 and 11-9)
Complete the sentences with *a/an, the,* or *Ø*.

**Online Security**

1. I got _____ email. _____ message asked me to call a number because they needed
   _____ my bank information. I didn't respond to _____ message.

2. Did you choose _____ password yet? _____ password you have is too short.

3. The email was _____ fake message because it had too many misspellings.

4. Do not put _____ personal information in a password.

5. _____ unknown hacker stole my personal information from _____ online company.

6. Hacking is _____ crime. _____ Hackers can end up in _____ jail.

**EXERCISE 38 ▶ Looking at grammar.** (Charts 11-8 and 11-9)
Complete the sentences with *a/an, the,* or *Ø*.

1. I have ____*a*____ window above my bed. I keep ____*the*____ window open at night.

2. Kathy likes to listen to _____ music when she studies.

3. Would you please turn _____ radio down? _____ music is too loud.

4. Last week I read _____ book about _____ life of Indira Gandhi, India's only female
   prime minister, who was assassinated in 1984.

5. Let's go swimming in _____ lake today. My cousins will be there.

6. When I was in Memorial Hospital, _____ nurses were wonderful.

7. I'm studying _____ grammar. I'm also studying _____ vocabulary.

8. This room is so hot, and I feel dizzy. I'm going outside. I need _____ air.

9. _____ air is humid today.

10. Ted, pass _____ salt, please. And _____ pepper. Thanks.

11. It was too cold to walk, so I took _____ taxi.

12. What a great dinner! _____ food was excellent — especially _____ fish. And _____ service was wonderful. Let's leave _____ server a good tip.

13. I can't get in _____ car. _____ doors are locked.

14. Liam isn't at _____ work. He stopped at _____ university to see his son.

**EXERCISE 39 ▶ Listening.** (Charts 11-8 and 11-9)
Listen to the passage. Then listen again and write **a/an**, **the**, or **Ø**.

Do you know these words?
- roof (of your mouth)
- nerves
- blood vessels
- swell up
- avoid

## ICE-CREAM HEADACHES

Have you ever eaten something really cold like ice cream and suddenly gotten _____ headache? This is known as _____ "ice-cream
<sub>1</sub> ... <sub>2</sub>
headache." About 30 percent of the population gets this type of headache. Here is one theory about why ice-cream headaches occur. _____ roof of your mouth has a lot of nerves. When
<sub>3</sub>
something cold touches _____ these nerves, they want to warm
<sub>4</sub>
up _____ your brain. Your blood vessels swell up, and this causes
<sub>5</sub>
pain. _____ ice-cream headaches generally go away after about
<sub>6</sub>
30–60 seconds. _____ best way to avoid these headaches is to
<sub>7</sub>
keep _____ cold food off _____ roof of your mouth.
<sub>8</sub> ... <sub>9</sub>

**EXERCISE 40 ▶ Warm-up.** (Chart 11-10)
Complete the questions with **the** or **Ø**.

*Would you like to see ...*

1. __the__ Andes Mountains?
2. __Ø__ Korea?
3. _____ Mexico City?

4. _____ Indian Ocean?
5. _____ Amazon River?
6. _____ Australia?

7. _____ Red Sea?
8. _____ Lake Michigan?
9. _____ Mount Fuji?

## 11-10 Using *The* or Ø with People and Places

| | |
|---|---|
| (a) We met Ø *Mr. Wang*.<br>I know Ø *Doctor Smith*.<br>Ø *President Rice* has been in the news. | **The** is NOT used with titled names.<br>INCORRECT: *We met the Mr. Wang.* |
| (b) He lives in Ø *Europe*.<br>Ø *Asia* is the largest continent.<br>Have you ever been to Ø *Africa*? | **The** is NOT used with the names of continents.<br>INCORRECT: *He lives in the Europe.* |
| (c) He lives in Ø *France*.<br>Ø *Brazil* is a large country.<br>Have you ever been to Ø *Thailand*? | **The** is NOT used with the names of most countries.<br>INCORRECT: *He lives in the France.* |
| (d) He lives in *the United States*.<br>*The Netherlands* is in Europe.<br>Have you ever been to *the Philippines*? | **The** is used in the names of only a few countries, as in (d). Others: *the Czech Republic, the United Arab Emirates, the Dominican Republic.* |
| (e) He lives in Ø *Paris*.<br>Ø *New York* is the largest city in the United States.<br>Have you ever been to Ø *Istanbul*? | **The** is NOT used with the names of cities.<br>INCORRECT: *He lives in the Paris.* |
| (f) *The Nile River* is long.<br>They crossed *the Pacific Ocean*.<br>*The Yellow Sea* is in Asia.<br><br>(g) Chicago is on Ø *Lake Michigan*.<br>Ø *Lake Titicaca* lies on the border between Peru and Bolivia. | **The** is used with the names of rivers, oceans, and seas.<br><br>**The** is NOT used with the names of lakes. |
| (h) We hiked in *the Alps*.<br>*The Andes* are in South America.<br><br>(i) He climbed Ø *Mount Everest*.<br>Ø *Mount Fuji* is in Japan. | **The** is used with the names of mountain ranges.<br>**The** is NOT used with the names of individual mountains. |

### EXERCISE 41 ▶ Game. (Chart 11-10)

Work in groups. Choose a place in the world. It can be a continent, country, city, sea, river, mountain, etc. Your classmates will try to guess where it is by asking *yes/no* questions. Try to limit the number of questions to ten for each place.

***Example:***
STUDENT A: (*thinking of the Mediterranean Sea*)
STUDENT B: Is it a continent?
STUDENT A: No.
STUDENT C: Is it hot?
STUDENT A: No.
STUDENT D: Is it big?
STUDENT A: Yes.
Etc.

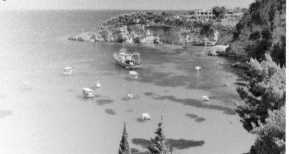

## EXERCISE 42 ▸ Game: trivia. (Chart 11-10)

Work in teams. Complete the sentences with *the* or Ø. Then decide if the statements are true or false. Circle "T" for true and "F" for false. The team with the most correct answers wins.★

1. _____ Moscow is the biggest city in _____ Russia.    T   F

2. _____ Rhine River flows through _____ Germany.    T   F

3. _____ Vienna is in _____ Australia.    T   F

4. _____ Yangtze is the longest river in _____ Asia.    T   F

5. _____ Atlantic Ocean is bigger than _____ Pacific.    T   F

6. _____ Rocky Mountains are located in _____

   Canada and _____ United States.    T   F

7. _____ Dr. Sigmund Freud is famous for his studies of

   astronomy.    T   F

8. _____ Lake Victoria is located in _____ Tanzania.    T   F

9. Another name for _____ Holland is _____ Netherlands.    T   F

10. _____ Swiss Alps are the tallest mountains in the world.    T   F

## EXERCISE 43 ▸ Game. (Chart 11-10)

Work in groups of 8-10 students. Each student says two sentences about two different places. One is true and one is false. Your classmates will guess which one is true and which one is false. Each correct answer is worth one point. If you use an article in your sentence incorrectly, you lose one point from your total. The student with the most points wins.

**Example:** I have hiked in the Alps. (*Students guess true or false.*)
I grew up in Kuala Lumpur. (*Students guess true or false.*)

## EXERCISE 44 ▸ Warm-up. (Chart 11-11)

Complete the sentences with information about yourself.

1. I was born in _____.
   (country)

2. I have lived most of my life in _____ .
   (continent)

3. This term I am studying _____.

4. Two of my favorite movies are _____ and

   _____.

---

★See *Trivia Answers*, p. 443.

## 11-11 Capitalization

**Capitalize**

| | | |
|---|---|---|
| 1. The first word of a sentence | We saw a movie last night. It was very good. | *Capitalize* = use a big letter, not a small letter |
| 2. The names of people | I met George Adams yesterday. | |
| 3. Titles used with the names of people | I saw Doctor (Dr.) Smith. There's Professor (Prof.) Lee. | I saw a doctor. BUT I saw Doctor Wilson. |
| 4. Months, days, holidays | I was born in April. Bob arrived last Monday. It snowed on New Year's Day. | NOTE: Seasons are not capitalized: *spring, summer, fall/autumn, winter.* |
| 5. The names of places: city state/province country continent | He lives in Chicago. She was born in California. They are from Mexico. Tibet is in Asia. | She lives in a city. BUT She lives in New York City. |
| ocean lake river desert mountain | They crossed the Atlantic Ocean. Chicago is on Lake Michigan. The Nile River flows north. The Sahara Desert is in Africa. We visited the Rocky Mountains. | They crossed a river. BUT They crossed the Yellow River. |
| school business | I go to the University of Florida. I work for the Boeing Company. | I go to a university. BUT I go to the University of Texas. |
| street building park, zoo | He lives on Grand Avenue. We have class in Ritter Hall. I went jogging in Forest Park. | We went to a park. BUT We went to Central Park. |
| 6. The names of courses | I'm taking Chemistry 101. | Here's your history book. BUT I'm taking History 101. |
| 7. The titles of books, articles, movies | *Gone with the Wind* *The Sound of the Mountain* | Capitalize the first word of a title. Capitalize all other words except articles (*the, a/an*), coordinating conjunctions (*and, but, or*), and short prepositions (*with, in, at, etc.*). |
| 8. The names of languages and nationalities | She speaks Spanish. We discussed Japanese customs. | Words that refer to the names of languages and nationalities are always capitalized. |
| 9. The names of religions | Buddhism, Christianity, Hinduism, Islam, and Judaism are major religions in the world. Talal is a Muslim. | Words that refer to the names of religions are always capitalized. |

**EXERCISE 45 ▶ Looking at grammar. (Chart 11-11)**
Capitalize the words in the sentences as necessary.

1. a. Do you know richard smith? He is a professor at this university.

   b. I know that professor smith teaches at the university of arizona.

2. a. I'm taking a history course this semester.

   b. I'm taking modern european history 101 this semester.

3. a. The amazon is a river in south america.

   b. The mississippi river flows south.

4. a. Canada is in north america.★

   b. Canada is north of the united states.

5. a. I find english grammar a little confusing.

   b. English grammar 099 is a difficult class.

   c. The title of this book is *fundamentals of english grammar*.

**EXERCISE 46 ▶ Looking at grammar. (Chart 11-11)**
Write "C" for correct and "I" for incorrect sentences. Add capital letters where necessary.

1. __I__ We're going to have a test next ᵀtuesday.

2. _____ Where was your mother born?

3. _____ John is a catholic. ali is a Muslim.

4. _____ Anita speaks French. She studied in France for two years.

5. _____ Venezuela is a spanish-speaking country.

6. _____ The sun rises in the east.

7. _____ We went to a zoo. My grandfather took me.

8. _____ On valentine's day (february 14th), sweethearts give each other presents.

9. _____ I read a book called *the cat and the mouse in my aunt's house*.

10. _____ We went to Vancouver, British Columbia, for our vacation last summer.

**EXERCISE 47 ▶ Check your knowledge. (Chapter 11 Review)**
Correct the errors.

1. Our teacher gave us a lot of new vocabularies to study.

2. Would you like to have little chicken and rice for lunch?

3. The school advisor had many suggestion for the student.

---

★When **north**, **south**, **east**, and **west** refer to the direction on a compass, they are not capitalized: *Japan is **east** of China.* When they are part of a geographical name, they are capitalized: *Japan is in the Far **East**.*

4. There is a urgent message for you to call the doctor.

5. My algebra 101 course is a fairly easy.

6. There were many interesting idea and strong opinion at the meeting.

7. My Father and I share the same Birthday.

8. What time did you feed a cats?

9. We're not going to order lunch. We just want coffee. Could we have two coffee, please?

10. Many students have trouble with a slang when they learn the English.

**EXERCISE 48 ▸ Reading and grammar.** (Chapter 11)
Read the passage. Add capital letters as necessary.

Do you know these words?
- recognize
- apes
- penny
- guidance
- trust
- observations

# JANE GOODALL

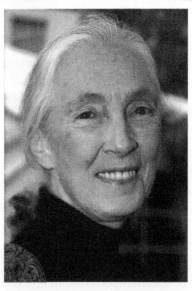

(1)   Do you recognize the name jane goodall? Perhaps you know her for her studies of chimpanzees. She became very famous from her work in tanzania.

(2)   Jane goodall was born in england, and as a child, was fascinated by animals. Her favorite books were *the jungle book*, by rudyard kipling, and books about tarzan, a fictional character who was raised by apes.

(3)   Her childhood dream was to go to africa. After high school, she worked as a secretary and a waitress to earn enough money to go there. During that time, she took evening courses in journalism and english literature. She saved every penny until she had enough money for a trip to africa.

(4)   In the spring of 1957, she sailed through the red sea and southward down the african coast to mombasa in kenya. Her uncle had arranged a job for her in nairobi with a british company. When she was there, she met dr. louis leakey, a famous anthropologist. Under his guidance, she began her lifelong study of chimpanzees on the eastern shore of lake tanganyika.

(5)   Jane goodall lived alone in a tent near the lake. Through months and years of patience, she won the trust of the chimps and was able to watch them closely. Her observations changed forever how we view chimpanzees — and many other animals we share the world with.

## EXERCISE 49 ▶ Reading, grammar, and writing. (Chapter 11)

**Part I.** Read the paragraph.

Do you know these words?
- roots
- shoots
- observe
- organization
- global
- deforestation
- service projects
- environment

# ROOTS AND SHOOTS

Jane Goodall went to Africa to study animals. She spent 40 years observing and studying chimpanzees in Tanzania. As a result of Dr. Goodall's work, an organization called Roots and Shoots was formed. This organization focuses on work that children and teenagers can do to help the local and global community. The idea began in 1991. A group of 16 teenagers met with Dr. Goodall at her home in Dar Es Salaam, Tanzania. They wanted to discuss how to help with a variety of problems, such as pollution, deforestation, and helping animals survive. Dr. Goodall was involved in the meetings, but the teenagers chose the service projects and did the work themselves. The first Roots and Shoots community project was a local one. The group educated villagers about better treatment of chickens at home and in the marketplace. Today, there are tens of thousands of members in almost 100 countries. They work to make the environment and the world better through community-service projects.

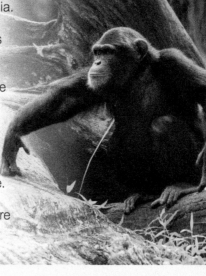

**Part II.** Choose the best description for each noun in green.

1. *chimpanzees*
   a. a specific group of chimpanzees in Tanzania
   b. not a specific group of chimpanzees in Tanzania

2. *the idea*
   a. a specific idea (work to help the local and global community)
   b. a non-specific idea (one idea among many)

3. *pollution*
   a. not specific (pollution around the world)
   b. specific (pollution in one place)

4. *the meetings*
   a. non-specific meetings
   b. specific meetings about a variety of problems

5. *the teenagers*
   a. a specific group of teenagers (16)
   b. teenagers in general

6. *the work*
   a. work in general
   b. specific work (service project work)

7. *the environment*
   a. one environment among many
   b. the environment we know, in our world

8. *the world*
   a. we know the world (the world we live in)
   b. one world of many

**Part III.** Write your own paragraph about an organization that is doing something to help people or animals. Focus on correct article usage and capitalization. Follow these steps:

1. Choose an organization you are interested in.

2. Research the organization. Find the organization's website if possible. Take notes on the information you find. Include details about its history, why it was formed, its goals and benefits, and the person or people who formed it. You can use the outline below as a model (add more capital letters if you have more than two details).

   I. History of the organization
      A.
      B.
  II. Purpose/goals of the organization
      A.
      B.
 III. Key people in the organization (if not already mentioned)
      A.
      B.
 IV. Results/Benefits of the organization
      A.
      B.

---

**WRITING TIP**

When you are taking notes from websites, books, or other media, write down the information in your own words. Don't copy directly from a source and present it as your own words. This is called *plagiarism*. Plagiarism is not acceptable in high schools, colleges, and universities.

Putting information in your own words also forces you to think about the meaning of the reading. This will help you understand and present the information more clearly.

Use the grammar you know. This will probably be simpler than how you write in your own language. If you try to write at a higher level before you are ready, you will probably translate a lot from your language into English. This can result in writing that has many errors.

---

**Part IV.** Edit your writing. Check for the following:

1. ☐ use of ***the*** for nouns with a specific meaning
2. ☐ use of ***a/an*** or **Ø** for nouns with a non-specific meaning
3. ☐ correct article usage for people and places
4. ☐ correct capitalization (review Chart 11-11)
5. ☐ the information is in your own words, not copied
6. ☐ correct spelling (use a dictionary or spell-check)

---

■■■■■ For digital resources, go to the Pearson Practice English app.

# CHAPTER 12

## Adjective Clauses

**PRETEST: What do I already know?**

Write "C" if the sentences are correct and "I" if they are incorrect.

1. _____ A teacher who is patient with students.  (Chart 12-1)

2. _____ The neighbor started her own online business has been very successful.  (Chart 12-1)

3. _____ I have a friend that recently got a part in a Hollywood movie.  (Chart 12-2)

4. _____ A friend whom I've known since childhood recently recommended me for a job.
(Chart 12-3)

5. _____ The movies that I enjoy the most have happy endings.  (Chart 12-4)

6. _____ Have you met the woman who are in your class?  (Chart 12-5)

7. _____ The hotel at which we are staying is offering the third night free.  (Chart 12-6)

8. _____ The host family Erik is living is very nice.  (Chart 12-6)

9. _____ The couple whose car died on their way to their wedding missed their flight for their
honeymoon.  (Chart 12-7)

**EXERCISE 1 ▶ Warm-up.  (Chart 12-1)**

Check (✓) the completions that are true for you.

*I have a friend who ...*

1. _____ likes to do exciting things.

2. _____ is interested in space.

3. _____ is studying to be an astronaut.

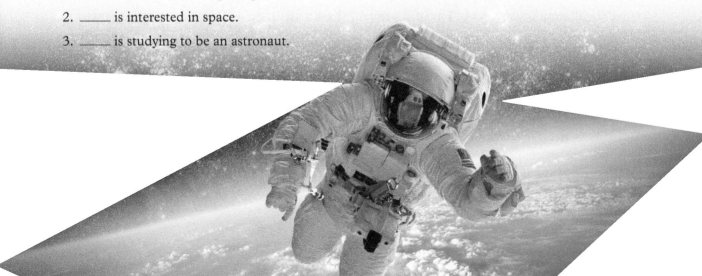

## 12-1 Adjective Clauses: Introduction

| Adjectives | Adjective Clauses |
|---|---|
| An ADJECTIVE modifies a noun. *Modify* means to change a little. An adjective describes or gives information about a noun. (See Chart 6-8, p. 171.) | An ADJECTIVE CLAUSE modifies a noun. It describes or gives information about a noun. |
| An adjective usually comes in front of a noun. | An adjective clause follows a noun. |
| (a) I met a [ADJECTIVE *kind*] + [NOUN *man.*] <br><br> (b) I met a [ADJECTIVE *famous*] + [NOUN *man.*] | (c) I met a [NOUN *man*] + [ADJECTIVE CLAUSE *who is kind to everybody.*] <br><br> (d) I met a [NOUN *man*] + [ADJECTIVE CLAUSE *who is a famous writer.*] <br><br> (e) I met a [NOUN *man*] + [ADJECTIVE CLAUSE *who lives in Oslo.*] |

### Grammar Terminology

(1) ***I met a man*** = an independent clause; it is a complete sentence.

(2) ***He lives in Oslo*** = an independent clause; it is a complete sentence.

(3) ***who lives in Oslo*** = a dependent clause; it is NOT a complete sentence.

(4) ***I met a man who lives in Oslo*** = an independent clause + a dependent clause; a complete sentence.

A *clause* is a structure that has a subject and a verb.

There are two kinds of clauses: *independent* and *dependent*.

- An *independent clause* is a main clause and can stand alone as a sentence, as in (1) and (2).

- A *dependent clause*, as in (3), is not a complete sentence. It must be connected to an independent clause, as in (4).

### EXERCISE 2 ▶ Looking at grammar. (Chart 12-1)

Check (✓) the complete sentences.

1. _____ I know a teenager. She flies airplanes.
2. _____ I know a teenager who flies airplanes.
3. _____ A teenager who flies airplanes.
4. _____ Who flies airplanes.
5. _____ Who flies airplanes?
6. _____ I know a teenager flies airplanes.
7. _____ I know a teenager who is a pilot.
8. _____ I know a teenager is a pilot.

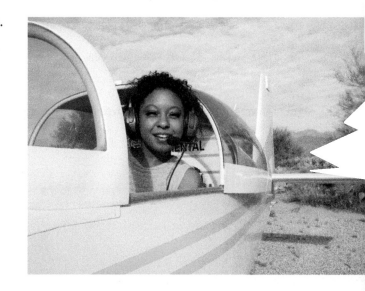

## EXERCISE 3 ▸ Warm-up. (Chart 12-2)

Complete the sentences with the correct words in the box. <u>Underline</u> the word that follows *doctor* in each sentence.

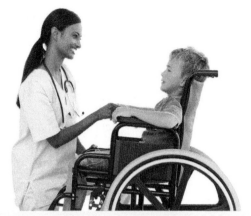

A dermatologist     An orthopedist     A pediatrician     A surgeon

1. _____ is a doctor who performs operations.

2. _____ is a doctor that treats skin problems.

3. _____ is a doctor who treats bone injuries.

4. _____ is a doctor that treats children.

---

### 12-2 Using *Who* and *That* in Adjective Clauses to Describe People

| | |
|---|---|
| (a) The man is friendly. <br><br> **s**   **v** <br> *He* lives next to me. <br> ↓ <br> *who* <br> ↓ <br> **s**   **v** <br> *who* lives next to me. | In adjective clauses, ***who*** and ***that*** are used as subject pronouns to describe people. <br><br> In (a): ***He*** is a subject pronoun. ***He*** refers to "the man." <br><br> To make an adjective clause, change ***he*** to ***who***. ***Who*** is a subject pronoun. ***Who*** refers to "the man." |
| (b) The man *who lives next to me* is friendly. | |
| (c) The woman is talkative. <br><br> **s**   **v** <br> *She* lives next to me. <br> ↓ <br> *that* <br> ↓ <br> **s**   **v** <br> *that* lives next to me. | ***That*** is also a subject pronoun and can replace ***who***, as in (d). <br><br> The subject pronouns ***who*** and ***that*** cannot be omitted from an adjective clause. <br><br> INCORRECT: *The woman lives next to me is talkative.* <br><br> As subject pronouns, both ***who*** and ***that*** are common in conversation, but ***who*** is more common in writing. |
| (d) The woman *that lives next to me* is talkative. | In (b) and (d): The adjective clause immediately follows the noun it modifies. <br><br> INCORRECT: *The woman is talkative that lives next to me.* |

## EXERCISE 4 ▸ Looking at grammar. (Chart 12-2)

<u>Underline</u> the adjective clause in the given sentence. Then change the given sentence to two shorter sentences with the same meaning.

**Rescuers**

1. The policewoman <u>who rescued the boy</u> was on her way home from work.
   a. _The policewoman rescued the boy_ .
   b. _The policewoman was on her way home from work_ .

2. The firefighter who answered the call broke a car window and rescued the injured person.
   a. _____ .
   b. _____ .

3. The EMT* restarted the heart of the man who collapsed at work.
   a. _____ .
   b. _____ .

4. The lifeguard who rescued the two swimmers had only been a lifeguard for one day.
   a. _____ .
   b. _____ .

5. The dog found the child who disappeared on a walk in the mountains.
   a. _____ .
   b. _____ .

## EXERCISE 5 ▸ Looking at grammar. (Chart 12-2)

Choose the sentences that express the ideas in the given sentence.

**The Vet**

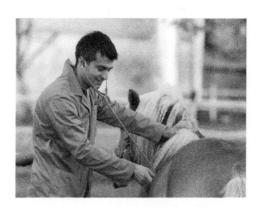

1. The veterinarian that took care of my daughter's pony is very gentle.
   a. The veterinarian is gentle.
   b. The veterinarian took care of a pony.
   c. The pony is gentle.
   d. The veterinarian took care of my daughter.

2. The veterinarian that treated our dog and cat recently passed away.
   a. The cat passed away.
   b. The veterinarian treated our dog.
   c. The veterinarian passed away.
   d. The veterinarian treated our cat.

---

*EMT = emergency medical technician

## EXERCISE 6 ▸ Looking at grammar. (Charts 12-1 and 12-2)

Underline each adjective clause. Draw an arrow to the noun it modifies.

**The People I Work With**

1. The assistant who manages the schedules speaks several languages.

2. The manager that hired me has less experience than I do.

3. I like the supervisor that works in the office next to mine.

4. My boss is a person who wakes up every morning with a positive attitude.

5. It's nice to work with people who have a positive attitude.

## EXERCISE 7 ▸ Looking at grammar. (Charts 12-1 and 12-2)

Combine each pair of sentences with **who** or **that**. The b. sentences will form adjective clauses.

**At a Restaurant**

1. a. Do you know the people?        b. They are sitting next to the window.

     _Do you know the people who/that are sitting next to the window?_

2. a. The manager was very friendly.    b. He took us to our table.

     _____

3. a. The server didn't write anything down.  b. She took our order.

     _____

4. a. The chef has won awards.       b. He makes the pasta.

     _____

5. a. My friends want to open another.   b. They run the restaurant.

     _____

6. a. I recognized a woman.        b. She was in my high school class.

     _____

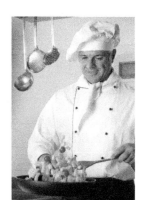

## EXERCISE 8 ▸ Let's talk. (Charts 12-1 and 12-2)

Work in pairs or small groups. Complete the sentences. Make true statements. Share some of your sentences with the class.

1. I know a man/woman who ...
2. I have a friend who ...
3. I like athletes who ...
4. Workers who ... are brave.
5. People who ... make me laugh.
6. Doctors who ... are admirable.

## EXERCISE 9 ▶ Looking at grammar. (Charts 12-1 and 12-2)
Add *who* or *that*.

**At a Swim Competition**

                   *who* **OR** *that*

1. I talked to the people ⌄ were in line with me to get tickets for the swim meet.

2. The swimmer had the fastest time was my cousin.

3. The man coached the visiting team was my teacher in high school.

4. The parents yelled at the swimmers were asked to leave.

5. I like to sit next to fans cheer the swimmers.

## EXERCISE 10 ▶ Warm-up. (Chart 12-3)
Complete the sentences with your own words.

1. The teacher that I had for first grade was _____.

2. The first English teacher I had was _____.

3. The first English teacher who I had wasn't _____.

| 12-3 | Using Object Pronouns in Adjective Clauses to Describe People |
|---|---|

|  |  |
|---|---|
| (a) The man was friendly.    S V O<br>     I met *him*.<br>     ↓<br>     *that* | In adjective clauses, pronouns are used as the object of a verb to describe people.<br><br>In (a): *him* is an object pronoun. *Him* refers to "the man."<br><br>One way to make an adjective clause is to change *him* to *that*. *That* is the object pronoun. *That* refers to "the man."<br><br>*That* comes at the beginning of an adjective clause. |
|         O    S V<br>(b) The man *that*   *I met*   was friendly.<br>(c) The man Ø    *I met*   was friendly. | An object pronoun can be omitted from an adjective clause, as in (c). |
|              S V    O<br>(d) The man was friendly. I met   *him*.<br>                      ↓<br>                      *who*<br>                      *whom* | *Him* can also be changed to *who* or *whom*, as in (e) and (f).<br><br>As an object pronoun, *that* is more common than *who* in speaking. Ø is the most common choice for both speaking and writing.<br><br>*Whom* is generally used only in very formal English. |
|         O     S V<br>(e) The man *who*    *I met*   was friendly.<br>(f) The man *whom I met*   was friendly. |  |

## EXERCISE 11 ▸ Looking at grammar. (Charts 12-2 and 12-3)
**Part I.** Check (✓) the sentences that have object pronouns.

**A Tech Repair**

1. _____ The technician that the company sent wasn't able to fix my Wi-Fi.

2. _____ The technician that came had just finished his training.

3. _____ The technician whom I spoke with asked his supervisor for help.

4. _____ The supervisor who arrived figured out the problem.

5. _____ The supervisor who the technician called was helpful.

6. _____ The supervisor who figured out the problem was very experienced.

**Part II.** Choose the correct word(s) for each sentence.

1. The tech ⟨who⟩/⟨whom⟩ I called wasn't able to help me.

2. The tech who / whom the company hired just graduated from high school.

3. The tech who / whom looked at my computer understood the problem immediately.

4. The tech who / whom reconnected my Wi-Fi worked very quickly.

5. The manager who / whom supervised the tech also came to my house.

6. The manager who / whom I contacted first had several suggestions.

## EXERCISE 12 ▸ Looking at grammar. (Charts 12-2 and 12-3)
Choose <u>all</u> the correct completions.

**Last Night's Party**

1. The man _____ teaches at a well-known cooking school.
   a. that prepared the food
   b. prepared the food
   c. who prepared the food
   d. whom prepared the food

2. A woman _____ has climbed Mount Everest.
   a. that I met last night
   b. I met last night
   c. who I met last night
   d. whom I met last night

3. The people _____ just moved into the neighborhood last month.
   a. that had the party
   b. had the party
   c. who had the party
   d. whom had the party

4. The friend _____ knew several people there.
   a. that I invited
   b. I invited
   c. who I invited
   d. whom I invited

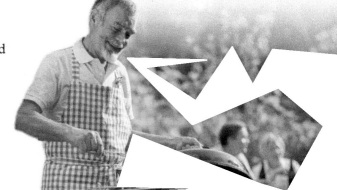

## EXERCISE 13 ▶ Looking at grammar. (Chart 12-3)

<u>Underline</u> the object pronouns in the b. sentences and change the sentences to adjective clauses. Use *that* or *whom*.

My Flight to New York

1. a. A woman snored the entire flight.      b. I sat in front of <u>her</u> on the plane.

   *A woman that/whom I sat in front of on the plane snored the entire flight.*

2. a. A man asked me for my phone number.      b. I hadn't met him before.

   _____

3. a. A woman had twin babies.      b. The flight attendant helped her.

   _____

4. a. A man tried to board early.      b. Security stopped him.

   _____

5. a. A man gave me his window seat.      b. I didn't know him.

   _____

## EXERCISE 14 ▶ Let's talk: pairwork. (Charts 12-2 and 12-3)

Work with a partner. Take turns making adjective clauses by combining the given sentences with the main sentence. Use *who*, *that*, or *whom*.

**Main sentence:** The man was helpful.
**Example:** He answered my question. → *The man who/that answered my question was helpful.*

1. He was working at the information desk.
2. I walked up to him.
3. I called him.
4. You recommended him.
5. He is the owner.
6. You invited him to the party.
7. He gave us a tour of the city.
8. I talked to him at the train station.
9. He sold us our museum tickets.
10. He gave me directions.

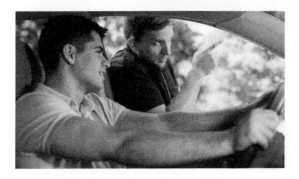

## EXERCISE 15 ▸ Looking at grammar. (Charts 12-2 and 12-3)
Complete the sentences with *that*, *Ø*, *who*, or *whom*. Write all the possible completions.

Family Connections

1. a. The man _____ married my mother is my best friend's uncle.

   b. The man _____ my mother married is my best friend's uncle.

2. a. The baby _____ my brother and his wife adopted was born to our cousin.

   b. The baby _____ was born to our cousin was adopted by my brother and his wife.

3. a. I don't know the cousin _____ is talking to Aunt Elsa.

   b. I don't know the cousin _____ Aunt Elsa is talking to.

## EXERCISE 16 ▸ Warm-up. (Chart 12-4)
Read the paragraph about James and then check (✓) the sentences that you agree with.
What do you notice about the adjective clauses in green?

Wanted: A Pet

James is looking for a pet. He is single and a little lonely. He isn't sure what kind of pet would be best for him. He lives on a large piece of property in the country. He is gone during the day from 8:00 A.M. to 5:00 P.M. but is home on weekends. He travels about two months a year but has neighbors that can take care of a pet, as long as it isn't too big. What kind of pet should he get?

1. _____ He should get a pet that likes to run and play, like a dog.

2. _____ He needs to get a pet which is easy to take care of, like a fish or turtle.

3. _____ He should get an animal that he can leave alone for a few days, like a cat.

4. _____ He needs to get an animal his neighbors will like.

5. _____ A pet that will talk to him, like a bird, is a good choice.

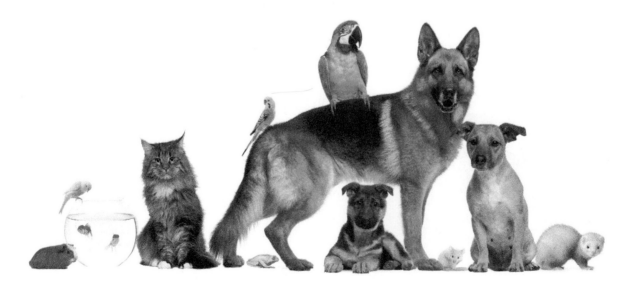

## 12-4 Using Pronouns in Adjective Clauses to Describe Things

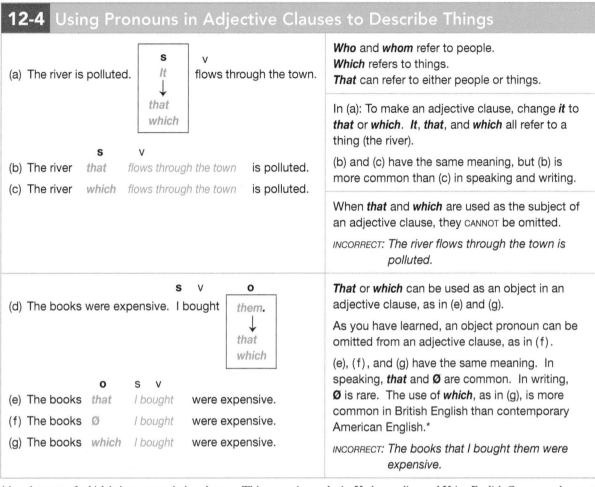

| | |
|---|---|
| (a) The river is polluted. **S** *It* **V** flows through the town. (→ *that* / *which*) | **Who** and **whom** refer to people.<br>**Which** refers to things.<br>**That** can refer to either people or things. |
| | In (a): To make an adjective clause, change *it* to **that** or **which**. *It*, **that**, and **which** all refer to a thing (the river). |
| (b) The river **S** *that* **V** *flows through the town* is polluted.<br>(c) The river *which* *flows through the town* is polluted. | (b) and (c) have the same meaning, but (b) is more common than (c) in speaking and writing. |
| | When **that** and **which** are used as the subject of an adjective clause, they CANNOT be omitted.<br>*INCORRECT: The river flows through the town is polluted.* |
| (d) The books were expensive. I bought **S V O** *them.* (→ *that* / *which*) | **That** or **which** can be used as an object in an adjective clause, as in (e) and (g).<br>As you have learned, an object pronoun can be omitted from an adjective clause, as in (f).<br>(e), (f), and (g) have the same meaning. In speaking, **that** and **Ø** are common. In writing, **Ø** is rare. The use of **which**, as in (g), is more common in British English than contemporary American English.* |
| (e) The books **O** *that* **S V** *I bought* were expensive.<br>(f) The books *Ø* *I bought* were expensive.<br>(g) The books *which* *I bought* were expensive. | *INCORRECT: The books that I bought them were expensive.* |

*Another use of *which* is in nonrestrictive clauses. This usage is taught in *Understanding and Using English Grammar,* the next level textbook in this series.

## EXERCISE 17 ▶ Looking at grammar. (Chart 12-4)
Underline each adjective clause. Draw an arrow from the adjective clause to the noun it modifies.

Lost and Found

1. The lost-and-found office <u>that we went to</u> was at the far end of the train station.

2. I left the scarf that I borrowed from my roommate on the train.

3. I turned in a cell phone that I found on my seat.

4. Some people post photos on social media of things that they find.

5. Lost items which are not claimed after 30 days are given

   to charity.

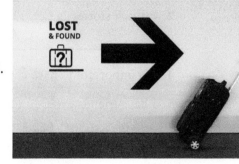

## EXERCISE 18 ▸ Looking at grammar. (Chart 12-4)

Combine each pair of sentences into one sentence. Give all possible forms.

Complaints

1. a. The pill made me too dizzy.
   b. I took it.

   _____The pill that / Ø / which I took made me dizzy._____

2. a. I bought a computer.
   b. It doesn't connect to the internet.

   _____

3. a. The clothes never came.
   b. I ordered them online.

   _____

4. a. The bus is usually late.
   b. It goes downtown.

   _____

5. a. I have a class.
   b. It has hours and hours of homework.

   _____

6. a. The soup was too salty.
   b. I bought it for lunch.

   _____

## EXERCISE 19 ▸ Looking at grammar. (Charts 12-2 → 12-4)

Complete the sentences with *who* or *that*. In some cases, both answers are possible.

What makes you "like" a video?

1. I "like" videos _____ make me feel hopeful.

2. I watch stories _____ are emotional.

3. People _____ make videos of their pets' funny behavior get a lot of "likes."

4. It's important to have clips _____ don't go on for a long time.

5. I have friends _____ think their lives are really interesting and film everyday
   activities. I don't "like" these videos.

**EXERCISE 20 ▸ Looking at grammar.** (Charts 12-3 and 12-4)
Cross out the incorrect pronouns in the adjective clauses.

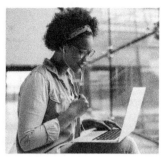

On Campus

1. The library I like to study in ~~it~~ is brand new.
2. The books I bought them at the bookstore were expensive.
3. I like the lunch special the cafeteria served it yesterday.
4. Professor Gomez is a teacher I would like to have him.
5. My roommate and I are really enjoying the TV that we bought it for our room.
6. The basketball player you see her on your way to class is an Olympic athlete.
7. The student center has a café that it serves wonderful coffee.
8. The coffee that the café serves it is organic.

**EXERCISE 21 ▸ Let's talk.** (Charts 12-2 → 12-4)
Work with a partner. Take turns making true sentences by using a word or phrase from each column. Use **who** or **that**.

| | | |
|---|---|---|
| | a person | |
| | people | works/work really hard |
| | students | relaxes/relax me |
| | parents | makes/make me happy |
| I know | grandparents | is/are interesting |
| I would like to meet | cousins | teaches/teach me a lot |
| I have | a pet | like/likes to have fun |
| I like | a co-worker | is/are surprising |
| | books | has an interesting life |
| | music | have interesting lives |
| | a hobby | is/are funny |
| | movies | |

**EXERCISE 22 ▸ Looking at grammar.** (Charts 12-2 → 12-4)
Cross out the words **who** or **that** where possible.

Help Desk

1. Tom called the help desk to talk with someone who could help with a password problem. (*no change*)
2. The manager ~~that~~ Tom called didn't know the answer.
3. The manager who helped Tom found the answer quickly.
4. The question that you asked is a common one.
5. The people who work in the office next door can help you.
6. The agent who my brother contacted put him on hold for twenty minutes.
7. I can find the information that you need.
8. The receptionist who I spoke with didn't understand my accent.

**EXERCISE 23 ▸ Listening.** (Charts 12-2 → 12-4)
Listen to the sentences. They all have adjective clauses. Choose the words you hear. If there is no subject or object pronoun, choose **Ø**. NOTE: In spoken English, *that* often sounds like "thut."

**My Mother's Hospital Stay**

*Example:* You will hear:    The doctor who treated my mother was very knowledgeable.

You will choose:  (who)    that    which    whom    Ø

| | | | | |
|---|---|---|---|---|
| 1. who | that | which | whom | Ø |
| 2. who | that | which | whom | Ø |
| 3. who | that | which | whom | Ø |
| 4. who | that | which | whom | Ø |
| 5. who | that | which | whom | Ø |
| 6. who | that | which | whom | Ø |
| 7. who | that | which | whom | Ø |
| 8. who | that | which | whom | Ø |

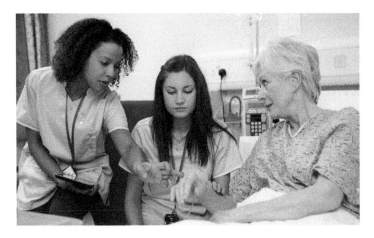

**EXERCISE 24 ▸ Let's talk.** (Charts 12-1 → 12-4)
Answer the questions in complete sentences. Use any appropriate pattern for the adjective clause. Use ***the*** with the noun that is modified by the adjective clause.

1. • One phone wasn't ringing.
   • The other phone was ringing.
      QUESTIONS: Which phone did Hasan answer? Which phone didn't he answer?
      → *Hasan answered **the** phone that was ringing.*
      → *He didn't answer **the** phone that wasn't ringing.*

2. • One student raised her hand in class.
   • Another student sat quietly in his seat.
      QUESTIONS: Which student asked the teacher a question? Which one didn't?

3. • One girl won the bike race.
   • The other girl lost the bike race.
      QUESTIONS: Which girl is happy? Which girl isn't happy?

4. • We ate some food from our garden.
   • We ate some food at a restaurant.
     QUESTIONS: Which food was expensive? Which food was inexpensive?

5. • One man was sleeping.
   • Another man was listening to the radio.
     QUESTIONS: Which man heard the special report about the earthquake in China?
                Which one didn't?

6. • One person bought a small car.
   • Another person bought a large car.
     QUESTION: Which person probably spent more money than the other?

**EXERCISE 25 ▶ Game.** (Charts 12-2 and 12-4)
Work in teams. Connect each phrase in the left column with the correct phrase in the right column.
Use **_that_** or **_who_**. Check your dictionary if necessary. The team that finishes first and has the most
grammatically correct sentences wins.

Definitions

***Example:*** 1. A hammer is a tool.
               g. It is used to pound nails.
               → *A hammer is a tool that is used to pound nails.*

1. A hammer is a tool. __g__

2. A comedian is someone. _____

3. An obstetrician is a doctor. _____

4. Plastic is a chemical material. _____

5. An architect is someone. _____

6. A puzzle is a problem. _____

7. A carnivore is an animal. _____

8. Steam is a gas. _____

9. A turtle is an animal. _____

10. A hermit is a person. _____

11. A pyramid is a structure. _____

a. She/He leaves society and lives
   completely alone.

b. He/She tells jokes.

c. It forms when water boils.

d. It is square at the bottom and has four sides that
   come together in a point at the top.

e. She/He designs buildings.

f. He/She delivers babies.

✓ g. It is used to pound nails.

h. It can be shaped and hardened to form many
   useful things.

i. It can be difficult to solve.

j. It eats meat.

k. It has a hard shell and can live in water
   or on land.

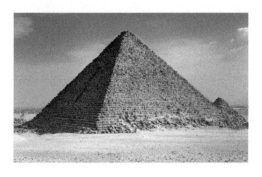

## EXERCISE 26 ▸ Warm-up. (Chart 12-5)

Read the sentences. What do you notice about the verbs in green and the nouns that precede them?

1. I have a friend who is vegetarian. He doesn't eat any meat.
2. I have friends who are vegetarian. They don't eat any meat.

| 12-5 Singular and Plural Verbs in Adjective Clauses | |
|---|---|
| (a) I know the man who is sitting over there. | In (a): The verb in the adjective clause (**is**) is singular because **who** refers to a singular noun, **man**. |
| (b) I know the people who are sitting over there. | In (b): The verb in the adjective clause (**are**) is plural because **who** refers to a plural noun, **people**. |

## EXERCISE 27 ▸ Looking at grammar. (Chart 12-5)

Choose the correct word for each sentence. <u>Underline</u> the noun that determines whether the verb should be singular or plural.

1. a. A saw is a <u>tool</u> that (cuts)/ cut   wood.

   b. Shovels are tools that   is / are   used to dig holes.

2. a. I am tutoring a student that   wants / want   to move to Montreal.

   b. Most people that   live / lives   in Montreal speak French as their first language.

3. a. I have a cousin who   climbs / climb   cell phone towers to repair them.

   b. People who   repairs / repair   cell phone towers can't be afraid of heights.

4. a. A professional athlete who   plays / play   tennis is called a tennis pro.

   b. Professional athletes who   plays / play   tennis for a living can make a lot of money.

5. a. Biographies are books which   tells / tell   the stories of people's lives.

   b. A book that   tells / tell   the story of a person's life is called a biography.

6. a. I sat next to some teens who   was / were   texting during a movie.

   b. A woman that   was / were   sitting near me complained to the manager.

## EXERCISE 28 ▸ Warm-up. (Chart 12-6)

Complete the sentences with your own words.

1. A person that I recently spoke to was _____ .

2. A person whom I recently spoke to wasn't _____ .

3. The room which we are sitting in is _____ .

4. The room we are sitting in has _____ .

5. The room in which we are sitting doesn't have _____ .

## 12-6 Using Prepositions in Adjective Clauses

| | | | | |
|---|---|---|---|---|
| | | **PREP** | **OBJ** | |
| (a) The man was nice. I talked | | to | him. | |

| | **OBJ** | | **PREP** | |
|---|---|---|---|---|
| (b) The man | that | I talked | to | was nice. |
| (c) The man | Ø | I talked | to | was nice. |
| (d) The man | whom | I talked | to | was nice. |

| | **PREP** | **OBJ** | | |
|---|---|---|---|---|
| (e) The man | to | whom | I talked | was nice. |

| | | **PREP** | **OBJ** | |
|---|---|---|---|---|
| (f) The chair is hard. I am sitting | | in | it. | |

| | **OBJ** | | **PREP** | |
|---|---|---|---|---|
| (g) The chair | that | I am sitting | in | is hard. |
| (h) The chair | Ø | I am sitting | in | is hard. |
| (i) The chair | which | I am sitting | in | is hard. |

| | **PREP** | **OBJ** | | |
|---|---|---|---|---|
| (j) The chair | in | which | I am sitting | is hard. |

*That*, *whom*, and *which* can be used as the object (OBJ) of a preposition (PREP) in an adjective clause.

REMINDER: An object pronoun can be omitted from an adjective clause, as in (c) and (h).

In very formal English, a preposition comes at the beginning of an adjective clause, followed by either *whom* or *which*, as in (e) and (j). This is not common in spoken English.

NOTE: In (e) and (j), *that* or *who* cannot be used, and the pronoun CANNOT be omitted.

(b), (c), (d), and (e) have the same meaning.

(g), (h), (i), and (j) have the same meaning.

## EXERCISE 29 ▸ Looking at grammar. (Chart 12-6)

Combine each pair of sentences. The b. sentence will form an adjective clause. Give <u>all</u> the possible forms of these clauses and <u>underline</u> them.

1. a. The movie was funny.                                   b. We went **to** it.

   → *The movie <u>that we went **to**</u> was funny.*
   → *The movie <u>**Ø** we went **to**</u> was funny.*
   → *The movie <u>which we went **to**</u> was funny.*
   → *The movie <u>**to** which we went</u> was funny.*

2. a. The man is over there.                                 b. I told you **about** him.

3. a. The woman pays me a fair salary.                       b. I work **for** her.

4. a. Alicia likes the family.                               b. She is living **with** them.

5. a. The job has 30 applicants.                             b. You are applying **for** it.

6. a. I enjoyed the music.                                   b. We listened **to** it in the car.

7. a. The class is closed.                                   b. The students want to sign up **for** it.

## EXERCISE 30 ▸ Looking at grammar. (Chart 12-6)
Complete the sentences with appropriate prepositions.* Draw brackets around the adjective clauses.

1. I spoke ___to___ a person. The person [I spoke ___to___] was friendly.

2. We went _____ a movie. The movie we went _____ was very good.

3. We stayed _____ a motel. The motel we stayed _____ was clean and comfortable.

4. We listened _____ a podcast. I enjoyed the podcast we listened _____.

5. Sally was waiting _____ a friend. The friend Sally was waiting _____ never came.

6. I talked _____ a clerk. The clerk _____ whom I talked was helpful.

7. I never found the book that I was looking _____.

8. The interviewer wanted to know the name of the college I had graduated _____.

9. My father is someone I've always been able to depend _____ when I need advice or help.

10. The person you waved _____ is waving back at you.

## EXERCISE 31 ▸ Looking at grammar. (Chart 12-6)
Complete each sentence with the information in the given sentence.

1. Oscar likes the Canadian family. He is staying with them this semester.
   a. Oscar likes the Canadian family with _whom he is staying_ this semester.
   b. Oscar likes the Canadian family that _he is staying with_ this semester.

2. This man is the manager. You should complain to him.
   a. This man is the manager who _____.
   b. This man is the manager to _____.

3. My sister is the person. I usually agree with.
   a. My sister is the person with _____.
   b. My sister is the person that _____.

4. The contract hasn't come. The lawyer is waiting for it.
   a. The contract that _____ hasn't come.
   b. The contract for _____ hasn't come.

5. Who is that person? You introduced me to him at the party.
   a. Who is that person that _____?
   b. Who is that person to _____?

---

*See Appendix Chart C-2 for a list of preposition combinations.

**EXERCISE 32 ▶ Listening.** (Charts 12-1 → 12-6)

Listen to the sentences and choose all the true statements.

*Example:* You will hear:   The university I want to attend is in New York.
       You will choose:   (a.) I want to go to a university.
              b.  I live in New York.
              (c.) The university is in New York.

1. a. The plane is leaving Denver.
   b. I'm taking a plane.
   c. The plane leaves at 7:00 A.M.

2. a. Stores are expensive.
   b. Good vegetables are always expensive.
   c. The best vegetables are at an expensive store.

3. a. My husband made eggs.
   b. I made breakfast.
   c. The eggs were cold.

4. a. I sent an email.
   b. Someone wanted my bank account number.
   c. An email had my bank account number.

5. a. The hotel clerk called my wife.
   b. The speaker spoke with the hotel clerk.
   c. The hotel room is going to have a view.

**EXERCISE 33 ▶ Reading and grammar.** (Charts 12-1 → 12-6)

**Part I.** Work in small groups. Answer the questions.

1. Have you visited or lived in another country?
2. What differences did you notice?
3. What customs did you like? What customs seemed strange to you?

Do you know these words?
- political views
- sense of humor
- appreciate
- have in common

**Part II.** Read the passage. Write the nouns that the pronouns refer to in the list on page 362.

**An Exchange Student in Ecuador**

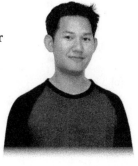

Hiroki is from Japan. When he was sixteen, he spent four months in South America. He stayed with a family who lived near Quito, Ecuador. Their
                                              1
way of life was very different from his. At first, many things that they did and
                                                                        2
said seemed strange to Hiroki: their eating customs, political views, ways of showing feelings, work habits, sense of humor, and more. He felt homesick for people who were more similar to him in their customs and habits.
          3

As time went on, Hiroki began to appreciate the way that his host family lived. Many activities
                                                             4
which he did with them began to feel natural, and he developed a friendship with each person in
  5
the family. At the beginning of his stay in Ecuador, he had noticed only the customs and habits
that were different between his host family and himself. At the end, he appreciated the many things
  6
which they also had in common.
  7

| | |
|---|---|
| 1. who  _____ | 5. which  _____ |
| 2. that  _____ | 6. that  _____ |
| 3. who  _____ | 7. which  _____ |
| 4. that  _____ | |

**Part III.** Complete the sentences with information from the passage.

1. One thing that Hiroki found strange _____ .

2. At first, he wanted to be with people _____ .

3. After a while, he began to better understand _____ .

4. At the end of his stay, he saw many things _____ .

## EXERCISE 34 ▶ Warm-up. (Chart 12-7)

Check (✓) all the sentences that are true about the given statement.

I spoke with a woman whose six children have won college scholarships.

1. _____ The woman has six children.

2. _____ I told a woman about my children.

3. _____ The woman told me about her children.

4. _____ Six children won scholarships.

5. _____ The woman received scholarships.

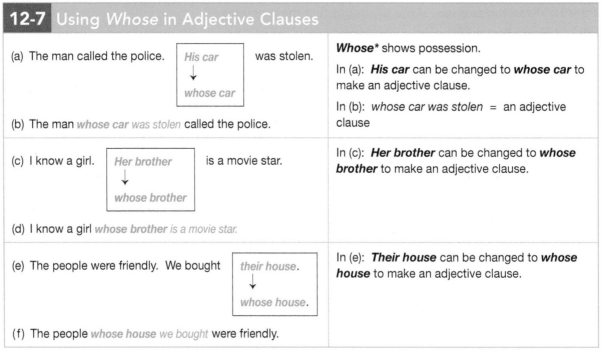

| **12-7** Using *Whose* in Adjective Clauses | |
|---|---|
| (a) The man called the police.  *His car* → *whose car*  was stolen.  (b) The man *whose car was stolen* called the police. | **Whose**\* shows possession. <br><br>In (a): **His car** can be changed to **whose car** to make an adjective clause. <br><br>In (b): *whose car was stolen* = an adjective clause |
| (c) I know a girl.  *Her brother* → *whose brother*  is a movie star.  (d) I know a girl *whose brother is a movie star.* | In (c): **Her brother** can be changed to **whose brother** to make an adjective clause. |
| (e) The people were friendly.  We bought  *their house.* → *whose house.*  (f) The people *whose house we bought* were friendly. | In (e): **Their house** can be changed to **whose house** to make an adjective clause. |

\***Whose** and **who's** have the same pronunciation but NOT the same meaning.
  **Who's** = **who is:  Who's** (*Who is*) *your teacher?*

## EXERCISE 35 ▸ Looking at grammar. (Chart 12-7)

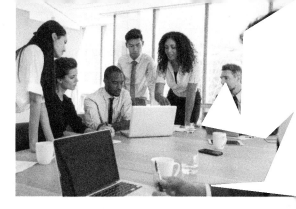

Combine each pair of sentences. Follow these steps:
  (1) Underline the possessive adjective in sentence b.
  (2) Draw an arrow to the noun it refers to in sentence a.
  (3) Replace the possessive adjective with **whose**.
  (4) Place **whose** + the noun that follows after the noun you drew an arrow to (in step 2).
  (5) Make one sentence by completing the **whose** phrase with the rest of the words from sentence b.

At Work

*whose*

*Example:* a. The woman is taking some time off from work.    b. Her baby is sick.
  → *The woman whose baby is sick is taking some time off from work.*

*whose*

  a. The man isn't worried.    b. You deleted his report.
  → *The man whose report you deleted isn't worried.*

1. a. The C.E.O.* is resigning.    b. His company lost money.

2. a. You should talk to the woman.    b. Her firm is hiring right now.

3. a. I spoke with some engineers.    b. Their department designs robots.

4. a. The manager is happy.    b. You edited his report.

5. a. A customer is on the phone.    b. We lost his order.

## EXERCISE 36 ▸ Grammar and speaking. (Chart 12-7)

Work with a partner. Take turns changing the b. sentences to adjective clauses by combining each pair of sentences with **whose**.

SITUATION: You and your friend are at a party. You are telling your friend about the people at the party.

1. a. There is the man.    b. His videos go viral.
   → *There is the man whose videos go viral.*

2. a. There is the woman.    b. Her husband writes movie scripts.

3. a. Over there is the man.    b. His daughter is in my English class.

4. a. Over there is the woman.    b. You met her sister yesterday.

5. a. There is the professor.    b. I'm taking her course.

6. a. That is the man.    b. His daughter is a newscaster.

7. a. That is the girl.    b. I taught her brother.

8. a. There is the boy.    b. His mother is a famous musician.

*C.E.O.* = chief executive officer or head of a company

## EXERCISE 37 ▸ Listening. (Chart 12-7)

Listen to the sentences and choose the words you hear: **who's** or **whose**.

*Example:* You will hear: The neighbor who's selling her house is moving overseas.
You will choose: (who's) whose

1. who's    whose
2. who's    whose
3. who's    whose
4. who's    whose
5. who's    whose
6. who's    whose

## EXERCISE 38 ▸ Grammar and speaking. (Chapter 12 Review)

Work in small groups. Change a. through f. to adjective clauses. Take turns completing each sentence.

1. The man _____ is an undercover police officer.
   a. His car was stolen.
      → *The man whose car was stolen*
        *is an undercover police officer.*
   b. He invited us to his party.
   c. His son broke our car window.
   d. His dog barks all night.
   e. He is standing out in the rain.
   f. His wife is an actress.

2. The nurse _____ is leaving for a trip across the Sahara Desert.
   a. Her picture was in the paper.
   b. Her father climbed Mount Everest.
   c. She helped me when I cut myself.
   d. She works for Dr. Lang.
   e. I found her purse.
   f. I worked with her father.

3. The book _____ is very valuable.
   a. Its pages are torn.
   b. It's on the table.
   c. Sam lost it.
   d. Its cover is missing.
   e. I gave it to you.
   f. I found.

## EXERCISE 39 ▸ Looking at grammar. (Chapter 12 Review)

Complete the sentences with all the possible choices: **who, that, Ø, which, whose,** or **whom**.

1. The family ___who / that___ moved into the house next door is from Kenya.

2. The mattress ___that / Ø / which___ I bought for my bed is comfortable but expensive.

3. Everyone _____ acted in the play enjoyed the experience.

4. Ms. Rice is the teacher _____ class I enjoy most.

5. The teen _____ I helped with his schoolwork got 100% on his exam.

6. I like the people with _____ I work.

7. I have a friend _____ father is a famous artist.

8. I recycled the cell phone _____ I replaced.

9. Students _____ have part-time jobs have to budget their time very carefully.

10. The man _____ car I dented was a little upset.

11. The person to _____ you should send your application is the Director of Admissions.

12. Some people believe almost anything _____ they see on the internet.

## EXERCISE 40 ▶ Listening. (Chapter 12 Review)
Listen to the conversation. Complete the sentences with *that*, *which*, *whose*, or Ø.

Friendly Advice

A: A magazine _____ I saw at the doctor's office had an article
<sub>1</sub>

_____ you ought to read. It's about the importance of exercise in dealing
<sub>2</sub>

with stress.

B: Why do you think I should read an article _____ deals with exercise and
<sub>3</sub>

stress?

A: If you stop and think for a minute, you can answer that question yourself. You're under a lot of

stress, and you don't get any exercise.

B: The stress _____ I have at work doesn't bother me. It's just a normal part
<sub>4</sub>

of my job. And I don't have time to exercise.

A: Well, you should make time. Anyone _____ job is as stressful as yours
<sub>5</sub>

should make physical exercise part of their* daily routine.

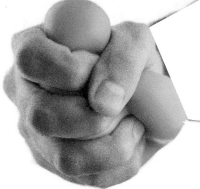

_____

*The use of *their* with *anyone* can be heard in informal English. In formal English, the speaker would say *his* or *her*.

**EXERCISE 41 ▸ Looking at grammar.** (Chapter 12 Review)
Complete the sentences by making adjective clauses from the statements in the box.

> it erupted in Indonesia in 1883
> its mouth was big enough to swallow a whole cow in one gulp
> their license plates have names instead of numbers
> ✓ it is chosen by most people for their car
> they can't jump
> they drink coffee six hours before their bedtime
> their specialty is brain surgery

Interesting Information

1. The color _that/which is chosen by most people for their car_ is silver.

2. People _____

   may reduce their sleep time by one hour.

3. Cars _____

   get noticed more.

4. Krakatoa, a volcano _____,

   caused temperatures to drop around the world.

5. Doctors _____ generally train for six to seven

   years after medical school.

6. Elephants are the only animals _____.

7. In prehistoric times, there was a dinosaur _____

   _____.

**EXERCISE 42 ▸ Let's talk: interview.** (Chapter 12 Review)
Ask two classmates each question. Share their responses with the class and see which answers are the most popular.

1. What is a dessert that you like? → *A dessert that I like is ice cream.*
2. What are some of the cities in the world you would like to visit?
3. What is one of the programs which you like to watch on TV?
4. What is one subject that you would like to know more about?
5. What are some sports you enjoy playing? Watching on TV?
6. What is one of the best movies that you've ever seen?
7. What is one of the hardest classes you've ever taken?
8. Who is one of the people that you admire most in the world?

**EXERCISE 43 ▸ Game.** (Chapter 12 Review)
Work in teams. Answer each question with sentences that have adjective clauses. The team that has the most grammatically correct answers wins.

*Example:* What are the qualities of a good friend?
→ *A good friend is someone who you can depend on in times of trouble.*
→ *A good friend is a person who accepts you as you are.*
→ *A good friend is someone you can trust with secrets.*
→ *Etc.*

1. What is your idea of the ideal roommate?
2. What are the qualities of a good neighbor?
3. What kind of people make good parents?
4. What are the qualities of a good boss and a bad boss?

**EXERCISE 44 ▸ Check your knowledge.** (Chapter 12 Review)
Correct the errors in adjective clauses.

1. The car that I bought it used to belong to my best friend.

2. The woman was nice that I met yesterday.

3. I met a woman who her husband is a famous lawyer.

4. Do you know the people who lives in that house?

5. The professor teaches Chemistry 101 is very good.

6. The people who I painted their house want me to do other work for them.

7. The people who I met them at the party last night were interesting.

8. I enjoyed the music that we listened to it.

9. The apple tree is producing fruit that we planted it last year.

10. Before I came here, I didn't have the opportunity to speak to people who their native language is English.

11. One thing I need to get a new hair dryer.

12. The people who was waiting to buy tickets for the game they were happy because their team had made it to the championship.

## EXERCISE 45 ▸ Reading and writing. (Chapter 12)

**Part I.** Read the passage and <u>underline</u> the adjective clauses. Read the passage again, but this time without the adjective clauses. Note the interesting information the adjective clauses add.

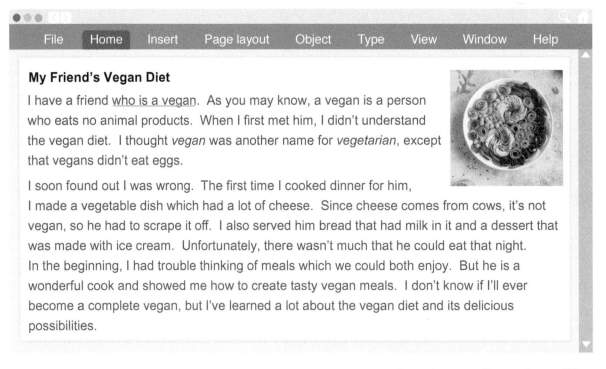

**My Friend's Vegan Diet**

I have a friend <u>who is a vegan</u>. As you may know, a vegan is a person who eats no animal products. When I first met him, I didn't understand the vegan diet. I thought *vegan* was another name for *vegetarian*, except that vegans didn't eat eggs.

I soon found out I was wrong. The first time I cooked dinner for him, I made a vegetable dish which had a lot of cheese. Since cheese comes from cows, it's not vegan, so he had to scrape it off. I also served him bread that had milk in it and a dessert that was made with ice cream. Unfortunately, there wasn't much that he could eat that night. In the beginning, I had trouble thinking of meals which we could both enjoy. But he is a wonderful cook and showed me how to create tasty vegan meals. I don't know if I'll ever become a complete vegan, but I've learned a lot about the vegan diet and its delicious possibilities.

**Part II.** Write a paragraph about someone interesting or unusual you know or know about. Use a few adjective clauses to add some interesting details.

*Sample beginnings:*

> I have a friend who ...
> I know a person who ...

---

### WRITING TIP

When you want to describe a person and include interesting or special information, first make a list of details to mention. Then put these details into a logical order. Next, decide how you can use adjectives and adjective clauses to add interesting and special information. Finally, write your description. Don't forget to have a topic and a summary sentence.

---

**Part III.** Edit your writing. Check for the following:

1. ☐ use of some adjective clauses
2. ☐ correct forms for the adjective clauses (***who, whom, which, that, whose, Ø***)
3. ☐ correct subject-agreement with adjective clauses
4. ☐ a topic sentence, details, and a summary sentence
5. ☐ correct spelling (use a dictionary or spell-check)

---

▪▪▪▪▪ For digital resources, go to the Pearson Practice English app.

# Gerunds and Infinitives

## PRETEST: What do I already know?

Choose all the correct answers.

1. Have you discussed _____ jobs with anyone yet? (Chart 13-1)
   a. to change          b. changing          c. about changing

2. We'll have a few hours before the train leaves. Do you want to _____? (Chart 13-2)
   a. sightseeing        b. go to sightseeing          c. go sightseeing

3. A new car is too expensive for Tom. He can't afford _____ one. (Chart 13-3)
   a. buy                b. to buy             c. buying

4. When the test was over, a few students continued _____. (Chart 13-4)
   a. to write           b. writing            c. to writing

5. Instead _____, let's walk to the mall. (Chart 13-5)
   a. of driving         b. driving            c. drive

6. Many people go _____ to the airport. (13-6)
   a. with the train     b. by a train         c. by train

7. It is hard _____ 100% on the driver's license test. (Chart 13-7)
   a. to get             b. get                c. getting

8. In many places, _____ drivers to text while driving. (Chart 13-8)
   a. it is illegal      b. is illegal for     c. it is illegal for

9. I ordered the clothes online _____ time. (Chart 13-9)
   a. to save            b. in order to save   c. saving

10. Are you _____ to sleep right now? (Chart 13-10)
    a. enough tired      b. tired enough       c. tired

## EXERCISE 1 ▶ Warm-up. (Chart 13-1)

Check (✓) all the completions that are true for you.

*I enjoy …*

1. _____ traveling.                3. _____ visiting tourist sites.

2. _____ going to museums.         4. _____ learning about ancient history.

## 13-1 Verb + Gerund

| VERB  GERUND<br>(a) I *enjoy walking* in the park. | A gerund is the *-ing* form of a verb. It is used as a noun.<br><br>In (a): ***walking*** is a gerund. It is used as the object of the verb ***enjoy***. |
|---|---|
| **Common Verbs Followed by Gerunds**<br>enjoy     (b) I *enjoy working* in my garden.<br>finish     (c) Ann *finished studying* at midnight.<br>quit     (d) David *quit smoking*.<br>mind     (e) Would you *mind opening* the window?<br>postpone     (f) I *postponed doing* my homework.<br>put off     (g) I *put off doing* my homework.<br>keep (on)     (h) *Keep (on) working*. Don't stop.<br>consider     (i) I'm *considering going* to Hawaii.<br>think about     (j) I'm *thinking about going* to Hawaii.<br>discuss     (k) They *discussed getting* a new car.<br>talk about     (l) They *talked about getting* a new car. | The verbs in the list are followed by gerunds. The list also contains phrasal verbs (e.g., *put off*) that are followed by gerunds.<br><br>The verbs in the list are NOT followed by *to* + the simple form of a verb (an infinitive).<br>    INCORRECT: *I enjoy to walk in the park.*<br>    INCORRECT: *Bob finished to study.*<br>    INCORRECT: *I'm thinking to go to Hawaii.*<br><br>See Chart 2-5, p. 43, for the spelling of *-ing* verb forms. |
| (m) I *considered not going* to class. | Negative form: ***not*** + *gerund* |

## EXERCISE 2 ▶ Looking at grammar. (Chart 13-1)

Complete each sentence with the correct form of a verb in the box.

| clean | ~~eat~~ | ~~hire~~ | sleep | work |
|---|---|---|---|---|
| ~~close~~ | hand in | pay | ~~smoke~~ | |

1. The Boyds own a bakery. They work seven days a week and they are very tired. They are thinking about ...

   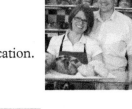

   a. ~~sleeping~~ *working* _____ fewer hours a day.

   b. *closing* _____ their shop for a few weeks and going on vacation.

   c. *hiring* _____ more workers for their shop.

2. Joseph wants to live a healthier life. He made several New Year's resolutions. For example, he will quit ...

   a. *smoking* _____ cigars.

   b. *eating* _____ high-fat foods.

   c. *sleeping* _____ until noon on weekends.

3. Martina is a procrastinator.\* She puts off ...

   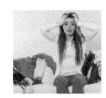

   a. *paying* _____ her bills.

   b. *handing in* _____ her assignments to her teacher.

   c. *cleaning* _____ her apartment.

---

\**procrastinator* = someone who postpones or delays doing things

**EXERCISE 3 ▸ Let's talk: pairwork.** (Chart 13-1)

Work with a partner. Complete each sentence with a gerund.

Looking Ahead

*Example:*

PARTNER A: It sounds like your aunt is becoming forgetful. Is she going to quit (*drive*) **driving**?
PARTNER B: Yes, she is going to quit **driving**.

| PARTNER A | PARTNER B |
|---|---|
| 1. Have you thought about (*take*) ____ some vacation time soon? | Yes, I've … |
| 2. It sounds like your apartment has a lot of problems. Have you considered (*move*) ____? | Yes, I've … |
| 3. Where's Martha? Has she finished (*study*) ____ yet? | No, she hasn't … |
| 4. Beth doesn't like her job. Is she talking about (*find*) ____ a different one? | Yes, she is … |

| PARTNER B | PARTNER A |
|---|---|
| 5. Jon and Cara fight a lot. Are they going to postpone (*get*) ____ married? | No, I don't think they are going to … |
| 6. Do you want to take a break, or do you want to keep on (*work*) ____ for another hour or so? | I think I want to keep on … |
| 7. I have a favor to ask. Would you mind (*drive*) ____ me to the doctor tomorrow? My car won't start. | No problem. I don't mind … |
| 8. You look tired. Are you going to put off (*study*) ____ for a few hours? | No, I can't put off … <br> *Change roles.* |

**EXERCISE 4 ▸ Listening.** (Chart 13-1)

Complete each short conversation with the words you hear. NOTE: There is a gerund in each completion.

*Example:* You will hear:  A: I enjoy watching sports on TV, especially soccer.
B: Me too.

You will write: I ___ *enjoy watching* ___ sports on TV, especially soccer.

1. A: Do you have any plans for this weekend?

   B: Henry and I _____ the dinosaur exhibit at the museum.

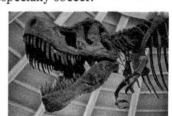

2. A: When you _____ your homework, could you help me in the kitchen?

   B: Sure.

3. A: I didn't understand the answer. _____ it?

   B: I'd be happy to.

4. A: I'm _____ the meeting tomorrow.

   B: Really? Why? I hope you go. We need your input.

5. A: I've been working on this math problem for an hour, and I still don't understand it.

   B: Well, don't give up. _____ .

## EXERCISE 5 ▸ Warm-up. (Chart 13-2)
Answer the questions.

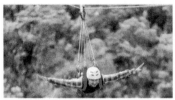

1. Have you ever gone ziplining?        yes      no

2. Would you like to go ziplining?      yes      no

| 13-2 | Go + -ing |
|---|---|

| | |
|---|---|
| (a) *Did* you *go shopping* yesterday? | **Go** is followed by a gerund in certain idiomatic expressions about activities. |
| (b) I *went swimming* last week. | NOTE: There is no **to** between **go** and the gerund. |
| (c) Bob *hasn't gone fishing* in years. | INCORRECT: *Did you go to shopping?* |

**Common Expressions with *go + -ing***

| | | | | |
|---|---|---|---|---|
| go boating | go dancing | go jogging/running | go sightseeing | go skydiving |
| go bowling | go fishing | go sailing | go (ice) skating | go swimming |
| go camping | go hiking | go (window) shopping | go (water) skiing | go ziplining |

## EXERCISE 6 ▸ Let's talk: interview. (Chart 13-2)
Make questions to ask your classmates about the activities. Use any appropriate verb tense. Share some of your answers with the class.

***Example:***  go waterskiing in the summer
> → *Do you go waterskiing in the summer?*
> → *Do you know someone who goes waterskiing in the summer?*
> → *Have you ever gone waterskiing in the summer?*

1. go skydiving
2. go bowling with friends
3. go dancing on weekends
4. go jogging for exercise
5. go fishing in the winter
6. go snow skiing
7. go camping in the snow

**EXERCISE 7 ▸ Let's talk: pairwork.** (Charts 13-1 and 13-2)
Work with a partner. Complete the conversation with each picture and the given information. Use expressions with **go + -ing** from Chart 13-2. Follow the model below. You can look at your book before you speak. When you speak, look at your partner.

A: Is/Are _____ here?

B: No, _____ isn't/aren't. _____ gone _____.

A: Oh, _____ often?

B: Yes, _____.

*Example:*

A: Is Sigrid here?

B: No, she isn't. She's gone skiing.

A: Oh, does she go skiing often?

B: Yes, she really enjoys skiing.

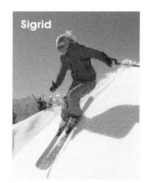

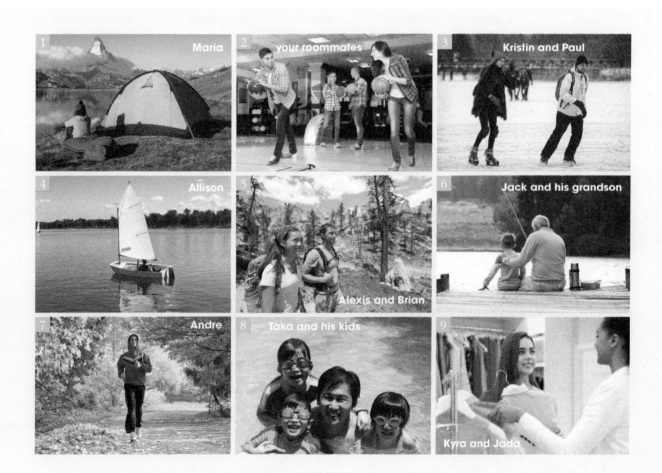

## EXERCISE 8 ▸ Warm-up. (Chart 13-3)

Check (✓) the sentences that are true for you.

1. _____ I hope to move to another town soon.

2. _____ I would like to get married in a few years.

3. _____ I intend to visit another country next year.

4. _____ I'm planning to become an English teacher.

## 13-3 Verb + Infinitive

| | |
|---|---|
| (a) Tom *offered to lend* me some money.<br>(b) I've *decided to buy* a new car. | Some verbs are followed by an infinitive.<br>Infinitive = ***to*** + *the simple form of a verb* |
| (c) I've *decided not to keep* my old car. | Negative form: ***not*** + infinitive |

**Common Verbs Followed by Infinitives**

| | | | | | |
|---|---|---|---|---|---|
| want | hope | decide | seem | learn (how) | can/can't afford |
| need | expect | promise | appear | try | can/can't wait |
| would like | plan | offer | pretend | be supposed | |
| would love | intend | agree | | | |
| | mean | refuse | | | |

## EXERCISE 9 ▸ Looking at grammar. (Chart 13-3)

Complete each sentence with the correct form of a word in the box.

| | | | | |
|---|---|---|---|---|
| be | ✓ fly to | hear | lend | visit |
| buy | get to | hurt | see | want |
| eat | ✓ go to | leave | tell | watch |

1. I'm planning ___*to fly to / to go to*___ Barcelona next week.

2. Hasan promised not _____ late for the wedding.

3. My husband and I would love _____ Fiji.

4. What time do you expect _____ our house?

5. You seem _____ that dress. Are you going to buy it?

6. Nadia appeared _____ asleep, but she wasn't. She was only pretending.

7. Nadia pretended _____ asleep. She pretended not _____ me when I spoke to her.

8. The Millers can't afford _____ a house.

9. My friend offered _____ me some money.

10. Tommy doesn't like vegetables. He refuses _____ them.

11. I try _____ class on time every day.

12. My wife and I wanted to do different things this weekend. Finally, I agreed

   _____ a movie with her Saturday, and she agreed _____

   the football game with me on Sunday.

13. I can't wait _____ my family again! It's been a long time.

14. I'm sorry. I didn't mean _____ you.

15. I learned how _____ time when I was six.

## EXERCISE 10 ▶ Let's talk: pairwork. (Chart 13-3)

Work with a partner. Take turns making sentences with a form of the given phrases. Use any appropriate verb tense.

*Example:* never learn how to use
PARTNER A: I will never learn how to use chopsticks.
PARTNER B: My grandmother has never learned how to drive.

1. promise to help
2. can't wait to see
3. hope to go
4. decide to try
5. plan to buy

6. can't afford to buy
7. need to finish
8. be supposed to write
9. mean to come
10. expect to get

## EXERCISE 11 ▶ Warm-up. (Chart 13-4)

Check (✓) the grammatically correct completions.

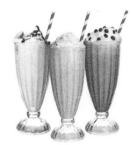

*Many children love ...*

1. _____ to drink milkshakes.

2. _____ drinking milkshakes.

3. _____ drink milkshakes.

---

### 13-4 Verb + Gerund or Infinitive

| | |
|---|---|
| (a) It *began raining*. <br> (b) It *began to rain*. | Some verbs take either a gerund, as in (a), or an infinitive, as in (b). Usually there is no difference in meaning. <br><br> Examples (a) and (b) have the same meaning. |

**Common Verbs That Take Either a Gerund or an Infinitive**

| | | |
|---|---|---|
| begin | like* | hate |
| start | love* | can't stand |
| continue | | |

*COMPARE: *Like* and *love* can be followed by either a gerund or an infinitive:
   *I like **going** / **to go** to movies. I love **playing** / **to play** chess.*

*Would like* and *would love* are followed by infinitives:
   *I would like **to go** to a movie tonight. I'd love **to play** a game of chess right now.*

## EXERCISE 12 ▸ Looking at grammar. (Chart 13-4)
Choose the correct verbs.

**Snow**

1. It started _____ around noon.
   a. snow         b. snowing         c. to snow

2. I continued _____ in the city.
   a. drive        b. driving         c. to drive

3. I don't like _____ out in the snow.
   a. be           b. being           c. to be

4. I would like _____ new snow tires for my car.
   a. get          b. getting         c. to get

5. My kids love _____ in the snow.
   a. play         b. playing         c. to play

6. They would love _____ near a big hill for sledding.
   a. live         b. living          c. to live

7. My parents hate _____ with icy sidewalks and roads.
   a. deal         b. dealing         c. to deal

8. They can't stand _____ the snow from their driveway and sidewalk.
   a. shovel       b. shoveling       c. to shovel

## EXERCISE 13 ▸ Let's talk: pairwork. (Charts 13-1, 13-3, and 13-4)
Work with a partner. Take turns combining the words in the box with the given phrases to make sentences about what you like and don't like to do.

| I like | I enjoy | I hate | I don't mind |
|--------|---------|--------|--------------|
| I love | I don't like | I can't stand | |

**Example:**   cook → *I like to cook. / I like cooking. / I hate to cook. / I hate cooking. / I don't mind cooking. / I don't enjoy cooking. / Etc.*

| PARTNER A | PARTNER B |
|-----------|-----------|
| 1. live in this city | 1. speak in front of a large group |
| 2. wash dishes | 2. travel by plane |
| 3. wait in airports | 3. wake up early |
| 4. go to parties where I don't know anyone | 4. listen to music while I'm falling asleep |
| 5. eat food slowly | 5. eat vegetables |
| 6. get in between two friends who are having an argument | 6. travel to unusual places |
| | *Change roles.* |

**EXERCISE 14 ▸ Grammar and speaking.** (Charts 13-1, 13-3, and 13-4)
Complete each sentence with the infinitive or gerund form of the verb in parentheses.
Then agree or disagree with the statement. Discuss your answers.

*What do you do when you can't understand a native English speaker?*

1. I pretend (*understand*) _____ .                                          yes    no

2. I keep on (*listen*) _____ politely.                                    yes    no

3. I think, "I can't wait (*get*) _____ out of here!" or         yes    no

   "I can't wait for this person (*stop*) _____ talking."          yes    no

4. I say, "Would you mind (*repeat*) _____ that?"                  yes    no

5. I begin (*nod*) _____ my head so I look like I understand.   yes    no

6. I start (*look*) _____ at my watch, so it appears I'm in a hurry.   yes    no

7. As soon as the person finishes (*speak*) _____, I say I have to leave.   yes    no

**EXERCISE 15 ▸ Looking at grammar.** (Charts 13-1, 13-3, and 13-4)
Complete the sentences with the infinitive or gerund form of the verbs in parentheses.

Roommates

1. I don't mind (*have*) _____ two roommates.

2. We like each other. We laugh a lot. The situation appears (*be*) _____ working.

3. We sometimes try (*eat*) _____ together, but we often don't finish

   (*cook*) _____ until around eight.

4. We are considering (*get*) _____ a TV.

5. One of my roommates has offered (*pay*) _____ for a satellite dish.

6. All of us hate (*wake up*) _____ early for morning classes.

7. The roommate in the room next to me is noisy in the mornings. I've quit (*set*) _____

   my alarm because she wakes me up.

8. A former roommate refused (*clean*) _____, so we asked her to move.

9. She also couldn't stand (*share*) _____ a bathroom.

10. We meant (*find*) _____ another roommate, but then we decided not to.

11. Our landlord seems (*want*) _____ (*raise*) _____ the rent.

    He keeps (*mention*) _____ it, but he hasn't done anything yet.

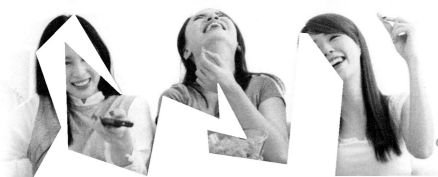

**EXERCISE 16 ▸ Let's talk: pairwork. (Charts 13-1 → 13-4)**
Work with a partner. Take turns completing the sentences with *to go*/*going* + *a place*.

*Example:* I would like ... .
PARTNER A: I **would like to go** to the Beach Café for dinner tonight.
PARTNER B: I **would like to go** to the movies later today.

1. I like ... .
2. I love ... .
3. I'd love ... .
4. I refuse ... .
5. I expect ... .
6. I promised ... .
7. I can't stand ... .
8. I waited ... .
9. I am thinking about ... .
10. Are you considering ... ?

11. I can't afford ... .
12. Would you mind ... ?
13. My friend and I agreed ... .
14. I hate ... .
15. I don't enjoy ... .
16. My friend and I discussed ... .
17. I've decided ... .
18. I don't mind ... .
19. Sometimes I put off ... .
20. I can't wait ... .

**EXERCISE 17 ▸ Looking at grammar. (Charts 13-1, 13-3, and 13-4)**
Complete the sentences with the infinitive or gerund form of the verbs in parentheses.
NOTE: When infinitives are connected by *and*, it is not necessary to use *to* with the second verb.

This Weekend

1. I want (*relax*) _____ this weekend.

2. I want (*stay*) _____ home and (*relax*) _____ this
   weekend.

3. I want (*stay*) _____ home, (*relax*) _____, and
   (*binge-watch\**) _____ movies this weekend.

4. Ella is thinking about (*get*) _____ up early in the morning and (*watch*)
   _____ the sunrise.

5. Ella is thinking about (*get*) _____ up early in the morning, (*watch*)
   _____ the sunrise, and (*sit*) _____ outside on her deck.

6. Mr. and Mrs. Bashir are discussing (*trade in*) _____ their old car and
   (*buy*) _____ a new one.

7. Kathy plans (*move*) _____ to New York City, (*find*) _____ a
   job, and (*start*) _____ a new life.

---

*\*binge-watch* = watch several episodes of a show or movie, one after another

8. Would you like (*go*) _____ out to eat and (*let*) _____ someone else do the cooking?

9. Kevin is thinking about (*quit*) _____ smoking and (*begin*) _____ an exercise program.

10. I'm planning to come to the office after you this weekend. Would you mind (*leave*) _____ the heat on but (*turn off*) _____ the lights and (*lock*) _____ the door?

## EXERCISE 18 ▶ Game. (Charts 13-1 → 13-4)

Work in teams. Your teacher will call out an item number. Make a sentence using the given words and any verb tense. Begin with **I**. The first team to come up with a grammatically correct sentence wins a point. The team with the most points wins the game.

***Example:*** want \ go
→ *I want to go to Dallas next week.*

1. plan \ go
2. consider \ go
3. offer \ help
4. like \ visit
5. enjoy \ read
6. intend \ get
7. can't afford \ buy
8. seem \ be
9. put off \ write
10. would like \ go \ swim

11. postpone \ go
12. finish \ study
13. would mind \ help
14. begin \ study
15. think about \ go
16. quit \ try
17. continue \ walk
18. learn \ speak
19. talk about \ go
20. keep \ try

## EXERCISE 19 ▶ Warm-up. (Chart 13-5)

Agree or disagree with the statements. Notice the use of the prepositions and gerunds in green that follow the verbs.

*I know someone who ...*

| | | |
|---|---|---|
| 1. never apologizes for being late. | yes | no |
| 2. is interested in coming to this country. | yes | no |
| 3. is worried about losing his/her job. | yes | no |
| 4. is excited about becoming a parent. | yes | no |
| 5. worries about his or her grades. | yes | no |
| 6. is looking forward to an exciting vacation. | yes | no |

## 13-5 Preposition + Gerund

| | |
|---|---|
| (a) Kate *insisted on coming* with us. | A preposition is followed by a gerund, not an infinitive. |
| (b) We're *excited about going* to Tahiti. | In (a): The preposition (*on*) is followed by a gerund |
| (c) I *apologized for being* late. | (*coming*). |

**Common Expressions with Prepositions Followed by Gerunds**

| | | |
|---|---|---|
| be afraid *of* (doing something) | apologize *for* | look forward *to* |
| be excited *about* | believe *in* | plan *on* |
| be good *at* | dream *about* / *of* | stop (someone) *from* |
| be interested *in* | feel *like* | thank (someone) *for* |
| be nervous *about* | forgive (someone) *for* | worry *about* / be worried *about* |
| be responsible *for* | insist *on* | |
| be tired *of* | instead *of* | |

## EXERCISE 20 ▸ Looking at grammar. (Chart 13-5)
Complete the sentences with the correct preposition.

1. Lyn ... moving.

    a. feels _____

    b. dreams _____

    c. is afraid _____

    d. is nervous _____

    e. is tired _____

    f. insisted _____

    g. plans _____

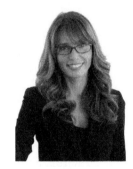

2. Sai is ... taking care of the kids.

    a. excited _____

    b. good _____

    c. interested _____

    d. looking forward _____

    e. planning _____

    f. responsible _____

    g. worried _____

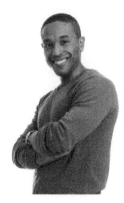

**EXERCISE 21 ▸ Looking at grammar. (Chart 13-5)**
Complete the sentences with a *preposition + gerund* and the given words.

1. I'm looking forward  +  go away for the weekend
   → I'm looking forward **to** *going away for the weekend.*

2. Thank you  +  hold the door open
3. I'm worried  +  be late for my appointment
4. Are you interested  +  go to the beach with us
5. I apologized  +  be late
6. Are you afraid  +  fly in small planes
7. Are you nervous  +  take your driver's test
8. We're excited  +  see the soccer game
9. Tariq insisted  +  pay the restaurant bill
10. Eva dreams  +  become a veterinarian someday
11. I don't feel  +  eat right now
12. Please forgive me  +  not get in touch sooner
13. I'm tired  +  live with five roommates
14. I believe  +  be honest at all times
15. Let's plan  +  meet at the restaurant at six
16. Who's responsible  +  clean the classroom
17. The police stopped us  +  enter the building
18. Jake's not very good  +  cut his own hair

**EXERCISE 22 ▸ Let's talk: pairwork. (Chart 13-5)**
Work with a partner. Take turns asking and answering questions using the following pattern:
***What*** + *the given words* + *preposition* + ***doing***.

*Examples:* be looking forward
PARTNER A: What are you looking forward to **doing?**
PARTNER B: I'm looking forward **to going to a movie tonight**.

　　　　dream
PARTNER A: What do you dream **about doing?**
PARTNER B: I dream **about becoming a professional athlete.**

| PARTNER A | PARTNER B |
|---|---|
| 1. be interested | 1. be nervous |
| 2. be worried | 2. be excited |
| 3. feel | 3. plan |
| 4. be good | 4. be responsible |
| 5. be afraid | 5. be tired |
| | *Change roles.* |

**EXERCISE 23 ▶ Listening.** (Charts 13-1 → 13-5)
Listen to the conversation. Then listen again and
complete the sentences with the words you hear.

**A Staycation**

A: Have you made any vacation plans?

B: Kind of. We're going to take a staycation.

A: You mean you're going to stay home and vacation?

B: Yeah. To be honest, I _____ so much.
      <sub>1</sub>

   I _____. It's so uncomfortable nowadays.
      <sub>2</sub>

A: But your wife _____, doesn't she?
                      <sub>3</sub>

B: Right. But we don't see our kids so much because they're in college. So we

   _____ time here so we can see them, and we can be tourists in
              <sub>4</sub>

   our own town.

A: So, what are you _____?
                        <sub>5</sub>

B: Well, we haven't seen the new Museum of Space yet. There's also a new art exhibit downtown.

   And my wife _____ in the harbor. Actually,
                          <sub>6</sub>

   when we _____ about it, we discovered there were lots of things to
                <sub>7</sub>

   do.

A: Sounds like a great solution!

B: Yeah, we're both really _____ our kids and more of our own town.
                              <sub>8</sub>

**EXERCISE 24 ▶ Looking at grammar.** (Chart 13-5)
Complete each sentence with the correct preposition and the gerund form of the verb in
parentheses.

1. Carlos is nervous ___*about*___ (*meet*) ___*meeting*___ his girlfriend's parents.

2. I believe _____ (*tell*) _____ the truth no matter what.

3. I don't swim in deep water. I'm afraid _____ (*drown*) _____.

4. I'm looking forward _____ (*take*) _____ a trip with my family.

5. Do you feel _____ (*tell*) _____ me why you're so sad?

6. My father-in-law insists _____ (*pay*) _____ when we go out for dinner.

7. I'm not very good _____ (*remember*) _____ people's names.

8. How do you stop someone _____ (*do*) _____ something dangerous?

9. The kids are responsible _____ (*take*) _____ out the garbage.

10. Monique lost her job. That's why she is afraid _____ (*have, not*) _____
_____ enough money to pay her rent.

11. Jo is pregnant and is looking forward _____ (*have*) _____ twins.

12. I sometimes (*dream*) _____ (*quit*) _____ my job, but instead _____
(*leave*) _____, I'll probably ask for a transfer.

## EXERCISE 25 ▸ Warm-up. (Chart 13-6)
Choose the completions that are true for you.

1. I sometimes pay for things _____.  a. by credit card  b. by check  c. in cash
2. I usually come to school _____.  a. by bus  b. by car  c. on foot
3. My favorite way to travel is _____.  a. by plane  b. by boat  c. by train
4. I communicate with my family _____.  a. by email  b. by text message  c. in person

## 13-6 Using *By* and *With* to Express How Something Is Done

| | |
|---|---|
| (a)  Pat turned off the TV *by pushing* the "off" button. | **By** + *a gerund* is used to express how something is done. |
| (b)  Mary goes to work *by bus*.<br>(c)  Andrea stirred her coffee *with a spoon*. | **By** or **with** followed by a noun is also used to express how something is done. |

**By Is Used for Means of Transportation and Communication**

| | | | |
|---|---|---|---|
| by (air)plane | by subway* | by mail/email | by air |
| by boat | by taxi | by (tele)phone | by land |
| by bus | by train | by fax | by sea |
| by car | by foot (*or:* on foot) | (*but:* in person) | |

**Other Uses of By**

| | | |
|---|---|---|
| by chance | by mistake | by check (*but:* in cash) |
| by choice | by hand** | by credit card |

**With Is Used for Instruments or Parts of the Body**
I cut down the tree *with an ax* (by using an ax).
I swept the floor *with a broom*.
She pointed to a spot on the map *with her finger*.

*\*by subway* = American English; *by underground, by tube* = British English.

\*\*The expression *by hand* is usually used to mean that something was made by a person, not by a machine: *This rug was made by hand*. (A person, not a machine, made this rug.)
COMPARE: *I touched his shoulder with my hand*.

## EXERCISE 26 ▶ Looking at grammar. (Chart 13-6)

Choose <u>all</u> the correct completions.

1. Oliver received the news by _____.
   a. mail
   b. email
   c. by an email
   d. mistake
   e. chance
   f. person

2. Christina ate her snack with _____.
   a. knife
   b. chopsticks
   c. a spoon
   d. a fork
   e. hand

3. Kevin cleaned the bedroom with _____.
   a. a broom
   b. hand
   c. a mop
   d. soap and water

4. Philippe went to the city center _____.
   a. by foot
   b. by train
   c. on foot
   d. by a car
   e. by taxi
   f. by bus
   g. by chance

## EXERCISE 27 ▶ Looking at grammar. (Chart 13-6)

Complete the sentences by using *by* + *a gerund*. Use the words in the box or your own words.

| | | | |
|---|---|---|---|
| eat | ✓memorize | take | watch |
| drink | smile | wag | wave |
| guess | stay | wash | |

1. Many students practice vocabulary _____*by memorizing*_____ words.

2. We clean our clothes _____ them in soap and water.

3. Khalid improved his English _____ a lot of TV.

4. We show other people we are happy _____.

5. We satisfy our hunger _____ something.

6. We quench our thirst _____ something.

7. I figured out what *quench* means _____.

8. Alex caught my attention _____ his arms in the air.

9. My dog shows me she is happy _____ her tail.

10. Carmen recovered from her cold _____ in bed and

_____ care of herself.

## EXERCISE 28 ▶ Vocabulary and speaking. (Chart 13-6)

**Part I.** Write the correct vocabulary word for each picture.

| | | | |
|---|---|---|---|
| a broom | a needle and thread | a saw | a spoon |
| a hammer | a pair of scissors | a shovel | a thermometer |

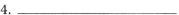 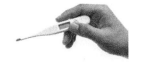

1. _____     2. _____     3. _____

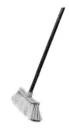 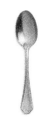

4. _____     5. _____

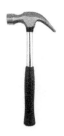 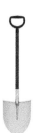 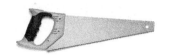

6. _____     7. _____     8. _____

**Part II.** Take turns asking and answering questions.

*Example:* clean the carpet
PARTNER A: How do you clean the carpet?
PARTNER B: I clean the carpet with a vacuum.

| PARTNER A | PARTNER B |
|---|---|
| *How do you ...* | *How do you ...* |
| 1. sweep the floor? | 1. eat soup? |
| 2. sew on a button? | 2. dig a hole in the garden? |
| 3. cut wood in half? | 3. nail two pieces of wood together? |
| 4. take your temperature? | 4. cut a piece of paper? |

## EXERCISE 29 ▸ Looking at grammar. (Chart 13-6)
Complete the sentences with **by** or **with**.

1. I opened the door ___*with*___ a key.

2. I went downtown ___*by*___ bus.

3. I dried the dishes _____ a dishtowel.

4. I went from Frankfurt to Vienna _____ train.

5. Ted drew a straight line _____ a ruler.

6. Rebecca tightened the screw in the corner of her eyeglasses _____ her fingernail.

7. I called Bill "Paul" _____ mistake.

8. I sent a copy of the contract _____ fax.

9. Talya protected her eyes from the sun _____ her hand.

10. My grandmother makes tablecloths _____ hand.

## EXERCISE 30 ▸ Warm-up. (Chart 13-7)
Read the passage and then agree or disagree with the statements.

### A White Lie

Rob gave his friend Paul a book for his birthday. When Paul opened it, he tried to look excited, but his wife had already given him the same book. Paul had just finished reading it, but he thanked Rob and said he was looking forward to reading it.

Paul told a "white lie." White lies are minor or unimportant lies that a person often tells to avoid hurting someone else's feelings.

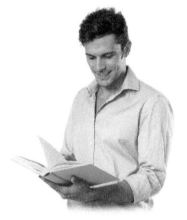

1. Telling white lies is common.            yes      no

2. It is sometimes acceptable to tell a white lie.   yes      no

3. I sometimes tell white lies.              yes      no

## 13-7 Using Gerunds as Subjects; Using *It* + Infinitive

| | |
|---|---|
| (a) *Riding* horses is fun. | Examples (a) and (b) have the same meaning. |
| (b) *It* is fun *to ride* horses. | In (a): A gerund (*riding*) is the subject of the sentence. |
| (c) *Coming* to class on time is important. | NOTE: The verb (*is*) is singular because a gerund is singular.* |
| (d) *It* is important *to come* to class on time. | In (b): *It* is used as the subject of the sentence. *It* has the same meaning as the infinitive phrase at the end of the sentence: *it* means *to ride horses.* |

*It is also correct (but less common) to use an infinitive as the subject of a sentence: *To ride horses is fun.*

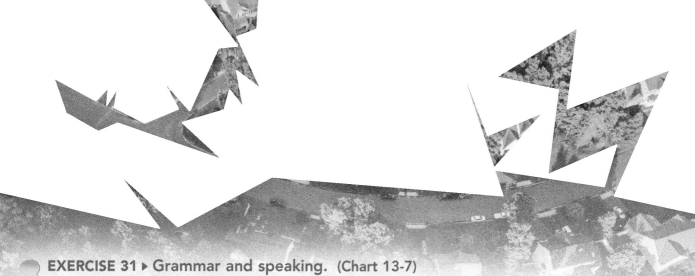

## EXERCISE 31 ▸ Grammar and speaking. (Chart 13-7)

Make sentences with the same meaning as the given sentences, and then decide if you agree with them. Circle *yes* or *no*. Compare your answers with a partner.

Living in This Town

**Part I.** Use a gerund as the subject.

1. It's hard to meet people here.

   → *Meeting people here is hard.*                    yes        no

2. It takes time to make friends here.                  yes        no

3. It is easy to get around the town.                   yes        no

4. Is it expensive to live here?                        yes        no

**Part II.** Use *it* + *an infinitive.*

5. Finding things to do on weekends is hard.

   → *It's hard to find things to do on weekends.*      yes        no

6. Walking alone at night is dangerous.                 yes        no

7. Exploring this town is fun.                          yes        no

8. Is finding affordable housing difficult?             yes        no

## EXERCISE 32 ▸ Let's talk: interview. (Chart 13-7)

Interview your classmates. Ask a question and then agree or disagree with your classmate's answer. Practice using both gerunds and infinitives in your answers.

*Example:*
STUDENT A (*book open*):   Which is easier: to make money or to spend money?
STUDENT B (*book closed*): It's easier to spend money than (it is) to make money.
STUDENT A (*book open*):   I agree. Spending money is easier than making money. OR
                           I don't agree. I think that making money is easier than spending money.

1. Which is more fun: to visit a big city or to spend time in the countryside?
2. Which is more difficult: to write English or to read English?
3. Which is easier: to understand spoken English or to speak English?
4. Which is more expensive: to go to a movie or to go to a concert?
5. Which is more comfortable: to wear shoes or to go barefoot?

6. Which is more satisfying: to give gifts or to receive them?

7. Which is more dangerous: to ride in a car or to ride in an airplane?

8. Which is more important: to come to class on time or to get an extra hour of sleep in the morning?

## EXERCISE 33 ▸ Warm-up. (Chart 13-8)

Agree or disagree with these statements.

*In my culture ...*

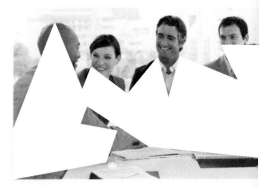

1. it is common for people to shake hands
   when they meet.                                    yes      no

2. it is important for people to look one another
   in the eye when they are introduced.              yes      no

3. it is strange for people to kiss one another
   on the cheek when they meet.                      yes      no

---

### 13-8  *It* + Infinitive: Using *For (Someone)*

| | |
|---|---|
| (a)  *You* should study hard.<br>(b)  It is important *for you* to study hard. | Examples (a) and (b) have a similar meaning.<br>Note the pattern in (b): |
| (c)  *Mary* should study hard.<br>(d)  It is important *for Mary* to study hard. | **It is** + *adjective* + **for** (someone) + *infinitive phrase* |
| (e)  *We* don't have to go to the meeting.<br>(f)  It isn't necessary *for us* to go to the meeting. | |
| (g)  *A dog* can't talk.<br>(h)  It is impossible *for a dog* to talk. | |

---

## EXERCISE 34 ▸ Looking at grammar. (Chart 13-8)

Complete the sentences with the given information. Use **for** (**someone**) and an infinitive phrase in each completion.

1. Students should do their homework.

   It's really important ___*for students to do their homework*_____.

2. Teachers should speak clearly.

   It's very important _____.

3. We don't have to hurry. There's plenty of time.

   It isn't necessary _____.

4. With final exams next week, I can't visit my sister this weekend.

   It's impossible _____.

5. Working parents have to budget their time carefully.

   It's necessary _____.

6. A young child usually can't sit still for a long time.

   It's difficult _____.

7. My family spends birthdays together.

   It's traditional _____.

8. My brother would love to travel to Mars someday.

   Will it be possible _____ to Mars someday?

9. I usually can't understand Mr. Alvarez. He talks too fast. How about you?

   Is it easy _____?

**EXERCISE 35 ▶ Reading and grammar.** (Charts 13-7 and 13-8)
**Part I.** Read the passage.

Do you know these words?
- handshake  - arm's length
- impolite  - universal
- rude  - cross-cultural
- varies  - gesture

# BODY LANGUAGE

Different cultures use different body language. In some countries, when people meet one another, they offer a strong handshake and look the other person straight in the eye. In other countries, however, it is impolite to shake hands firmly, and it is equally rude to look a person in the eye.

The distance that people stand when they talk to one another varies from country to country. In the United States and Canada, people prefer standing just a little less than an arm's length from someone. But many people in the Middle East and Latin America like moving in closer during a conversation.

Smiling at another person is a universal, cross-cultural gesture. Although people may smile more frequently in some countries than in others, people around the world understand the meaning of a smile.

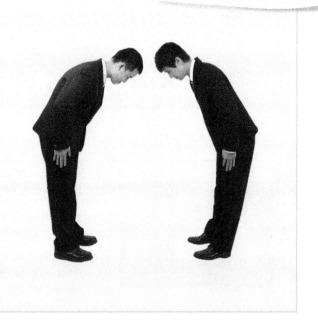

**Part II.** Complete the sentences with information about body language.

1. In some countries, it is important _____.

2. In some countries, _____ is impolite.

3. In my country, _____ is important.

4. In my country, it is impolite _____.

**EXERCISE 36 ▶ Let's talk.** (Charts 13-7 and 13-8)

In small groups, make sentences by combining the words in the box with the given phrases. Use gerunds as subjects or *it* + *an infinitive*. Share some sentences for other groups to agree or disagree with.

| | | | | |
|---|---|---|---|---|
| boring | embarrassing | hard | impossible | scary |
| dangerous | exciting | illegal | interesting | a waste of time |
| educational | fun | important | relaxing | |

*Example:* ride a bike

> → *Riding a bike is fun.* OR *It's fun to ride a bike.*

1. ride a roller coaster
2. read newspapers
3. study economics
4. drive ten miles over the speed limit
5. walk in a cemetery at night
6. know the meaning of every word in a dictionary
7. never tell a lie
8. visit museums
9. play video games all day

**EXERCISE 37 ▶ Reading and grammar.** (Charts 13-1 and 13-3 → 13-8)

**Part I.** Read the blog entry by co-author Stacy Hagen. Note the gerunds and infinitives in green. With a partner, explain why a gerund or infinitive is used.

Do you know these words?
- casual
- challenging
- acceptable
- politics
- likely

## BlackBookBlog

### Service with a Smile

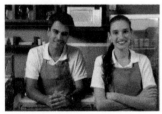

When you are a customer in a store or restaurant, how do you feel when an employee smiles at you? For example, let's say you are ordering a meal, and the server is very friendly and smiles a lot. Does it feel normal or strange to see such behavior?

In some cultures, as in the United States, customers expect it. It's called "service with a smile." It is important for employees to smile when they deal with the public.

Part of this expectation is also eye contact. Employees are supposed to look directly at the customer when they speak with them. Looking away is considered rude.

Imagine you are a cashier at a store right now, and you are taking a customer's money. How comfortable are you with the idea of smiling? What about looking directly at the customer?

If you are going to choose a job where you are expected to provide service with a smile, it is good to practice both eye contact and smiling until they come naturally to you. Your customer will expect you to do it, and your manager will be happier.

**Part II.** Agree or disagree with the statements. Discuss your answers with the class.

*In my country, …*

|   |   |   |   |
|---|---|---|---|
| 1. it is natural to smile a lot at people. | yes | no |
| 2. smiling a lot is too friendly. | yes | no |
| 3. looking directly at someone is rude. | yes | no |
| 4. customer service includes smiling at customers. | yes | no |
| 5. customer service includes looking directly at customers. | yes | no |

## EXERCISE 38 ▶ Warm-up. (Chart 13-9)

Check (✓) all the sentences that are grammatically correct.

1. _____ I went to the pharmacy because I wanted to pick up a prescription.

2. _____ I went to the pharmacy in order to pick up a prescription.

3. _____ I went to the pharmacy to pick up a prescription.

4. _____ I went to the pharmacy for a prescription.

5. _____ I went to the pharmacy for to pick up a prescription.

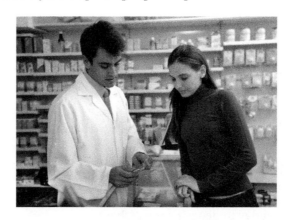

| 13-9 | Expressing Purpose with *In Order To* and *For* | |
|---|---|---|
| — *Why did you go to the post office?*<br>(a)  I went to the post office *because I wanted to mail a letter.*<br>(b)  I went to the post office *in order to mail a letter.*<br>(c)  I went to the post office *to mail a letter.* | ***In order to*** expresses purpose. It answers the question "Why?"<br><br>In (c): ***in order*** is frequently omitted. Examples (a), (b), and (c) have the same meaning. |
| (d)  I went to the post office *for some stamps.*<br>(e)  I went to the post office *to buy some stamps.*<br>    INCORRECT: *I went to the post office for to buy some stamps.*<br>    INCORRECT: *I went to the post office for buying some stamps.* | ***For*** is also used to express purpose, but it is a preposition and is followed by a noun phrase, as in (d). |

**EXERCISE 39 ▸ Looking at grammar.** (Chart 13-9)
Make sentences by combining the phrases in the left column with those in the right column.
Connect the ideas with (*in order*) *to*. Take turns saying the sentences with a partner.

*Example:* I called the hotel desk _____.
→ *I called the hotel desk (in order) to ask for an extra pillow.*

1. I called the hotel desk __e__.
2. I turned on the radio _____.
3. Nick went to Nepal _____.
4. People wear boots _____.
5. I looked on the internet _____.
6. Ms. Lane stood on her tiptoes _____.
7. The dentist moved the light closer to my face _____.
8. I clapped my hands and yelled _____.
9. Maria took a walk in the park _____.
10. I offered my cousin some money _____.

a. keep their feet warm and dry
b. reach the top shelf
c. listen to a baseball game
d. find the population of Malaysia
✓e. ask for an extra pillow
f. chase a mean dog away
g. help her pay the rent
h. get some fresh air and exercise
i. climb Mount Everest
j. look into my mouth

**EXERCISE 40 ▸ Looking at grammar.** (Chart 13-9)
Add *in order* to the sentences where possible.

1. I went to the bank to cash a check.
    → *I went to the bank in order to cash a check.*

2. I'd like to see that movie.
    → *(No change.)*

3. Sam went to the hospital to visit a friend.

4. I need to go to the bank today.

5. I need to go to the bank today to deposit my paycheck.

6. On my way home, I stopped at the store to buy some shampoo.

7. Masako went to the cafeteria to eat lunch.

8. Jack and Katya have decided to get married.

9. Pedro watches TV to improve his English.

10. I didn't forget to pay my rent.

11. Donna expects to graduate next spring.

12. Jerry needs to go to the bookstore to buy school supplies.

13. Mira hopes to complete college with a double major in physics and biology.

14. Hector asked to leave early for a doctor's appointment.

## EXERCISE 41 ▶ Looking at grammar. (Chart 13-9)

Complete the sentences with *to* or *for*.

Moving to Chicago

1. I moved to Chicago ___*for*___ my education.

2. I wanted to live in the city ___*to*___ attend graduate school.

3. I needed to leave my family _____ graduate school.

4. I decided to attend graduate school _____ get a good job.

5. I like to take long walks along the lakeshore _____ relax.

6. I take long walks along the lakeshore _____ relaxation.

7. In the winter, I wear a heavy coat _____ protect myself from the wind and cold.

8. I take the train to school _____ have more time to study.

9. I go to the Art Institute of Chicago _____ fun.

10. I like to go out _____ eat Chicago-style pizza.

## EXERCISE 42 ▶ Reading and grammar. (Charts 13-1 and 13-3 → 13-9)

**Part I.** Read the passage.

# CAR SHARING

Do you know these words?
- fee
- rate
- available
- maintenance costs
- members
- effective alternative
- parking lot

In hundreds of cities around the world, people can use a car without actually owning one. It's known as car sharing.

Car sharing works like this: people pay a fee to join a car-sharing organization. These organizations have cars available in different parts of a city 24 hours a day. Members make reservations for a car and then go to one of several parking lots in the city to pick up the car. They pay an hourly or daily rate for driving it. They may also pay a charge for every mile/kilometer they drive. When they are finished, they return the car to a parking area for someone else to use.

Car sharing works well for several reasons. Some people only need to drive occasionally. Oftentimes, people only need a car for special occasions like moving items or taking long trips. Many people don't want the costs or responsibilities of owning a car. The car-sharing organization pays for gas, insurance, cleaning, and maintenance costs. Members also don't have to wait in line or fill out forms in order to get a car. They know a variety of cars will be available when they need one.

Car sharing also benefits the environment. People drive only when they need to, and fewer cars on the road means less traffic and pollution. As more cities become interested in reducing traffic, car-sharing programs are becoming an effective alternative to owning a car.

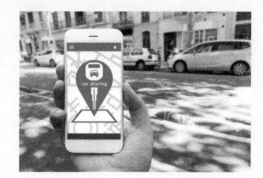

**Part II.** Complete the sentences with information from Part I. Use gerunds or infinitives.

1. _____ is helpful to people who don't own a car.

2. People pay a fee in order _____ a car-sharing organization.

3. Car-sharing members pay an hourly or daily rate for _____ a car.

4. Sometimes people need a car to _____ furniture or to _____ a trip.

5. Many people don't want the costs of _____ a car.

6. Cities are interested in _____ traffic.

**EXERCISE 43 ▸ Warm-up: pairwork.** (Charts 13-10)
Work with a partner. Read the conversation aloud and complete the sentences with the correct words in the box.

| strong | heavy | strength |

PARTNER A: Can you pick up a piano?

PARTNER B: No. It's too _____ for me to pick up.
        <sub>1</sub>
How about you? Can you pick up a piano?

PARTNER A: No, I'm not _____ enough to pick
        <sub>2</sub>
one up. What about the class? Can we pick up a piano together?

PARTNER B: Maybe. We might have enough _____ to do that as a class.
        <sub>3</sub>

---

## 13-10 Using Infinitives with *Too* and *Enough*

| | | | | | Infinitives often follow expressions with **too**. |
|---|---|---|---|---|---|
| | TOO + ADJECTIVE + (FOR SOMEONE) + INFINITIVE | | | | **Too** comes in front of an adjective. In the speaker's mind, the use of **too** implies a negative result. |
| (a) That box is | *too heavy* | | *to lift.* | | |
| (b) A piano is | *too heavy* | *for me* | *to lift.* | | |
| (c) That box is | *too heavy* | *for Bob* | *to lift.* | | |
| | ENOUGH + NOUN + INFINITIVE | | | | COMPARE: |
| (d) I don't have | *enough money* | | *to buy* that car. | | *The box is too heavy. I can't lift it.* |
| (e) Did you have | *enough time* | | *to finish* the test? | | *The box is very heavy, but I can lift it.* |
| | ADJECTIVE + ENOUGH + INFINITIVE | | | | Infinitives often follow expressions with **enough.** |
| (f) Jimmy isn't | *old enough* | | *to go* to school. | | **Enough** comes in front of a noun.* |
| (g) Are you | *hungry enough* | | *to eat* three sandwiches? | | **Enough** follows an adjective. |

*__Enough__ can also follow a noun: *I don't have **money enough** to buy that car.* In everyday English, however, __enough__ usually comes in front of a noun.

**EXERCISE 44 ▸ Looking at grammar.** (Chart 13-10)
Look at each picture and complete the sentences. Use *too* or *enough* + *an infinitive*.

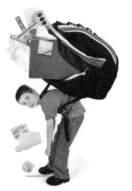

Picture 1

1. a. *heavy / carry*    The backpack is _____ *too heavy* _____ for the boy _____ *to carry* _____ .

   b. *strong / carry*    The boy is not _*strong enough to carry*_ the backpack.

   c. *big / carry*    The backpack is not _____ all his things.

   d. *small / carry*    The boy is _____ the backpack.

   e. *full / carry*    The backpack is _____ more things.

   f. *old / carry*    Is the boy _____ such a heavy backpack?

   g. *young / carry*    Is the boy _____ such a heavy backpack?

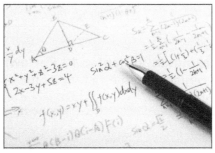

Picture 2

2. a. *complicated / understand*    The problem is _____ .

   b. *smart / figure out*    The student doesn't feel _____ the problem.

   c. *hard / figure out*    Is the problem _____ for the student _____ _____ ?

   d. *clear / understand*    The explanation isn't _____ _____ .

## EXERCISE 45 ▶ Looking at grammar. (Chart 13-10)

**Part I.** Combine each pair of sentences with *too*.

1. We can't go swimming today. It's very cold.
   → *It's too cold (for us) to go swimming today.*
2. I couldn't finish my homework last night. I was very sleepy.
3. Mike couldn't go to his aunt's housewarming party. He was very busy.
4. This jacket is very small. I can't wear it.
5. I live far from school. I can't walk there.

**Part II.** Combine each pair of sentences with *enough*.

6. I can't reach the top shelf. I'm not that tall.
   → *I'm not tall enough to reach the top shelf.*
7. I can't move this furniture. I'm not very strong.
8. It's not warm today. You can't go outside without a coat.
9. I didn't stay home and miss work. I wasn't really sick, but I didn't feel good all day.

## EXERCISE 46 ▶ Let's talk: pairwork. (Chart 13-10)

Work with a partner. Take turns completing the sentences with infinitives.

| PARTNER A | PARTNER B |
|---|---|
| 1. I'm too short … . | 6. A sports car is too expensive … . |
| 2. I'm not tall enough … . | 7. I don't have enough money … . |
| 3. I'm not strong enough … . | 8. Yesterday I didn't have enough time … . |
| 4. Last night I was too tired … . | 9. A teenager is old enough … but too young … . |
| 5. Yesterday I was too busy … . | 10. I know enough English … but not enough … . |
| | *Change roles.* |

## EXERCISE 47 ▶ Looking at grammar. (Chapter 13 Review)

Complete each sentence with the gerund or infinitive form of the word in parentheses.

1. It's difficult for me (*remember*) ___to remember___ phone numbers.

2. My cat is good at (*catch*) ___catching___ mice.

3. I called my friend (*invite*) _____ her for dinner.

4. Fatima talked about (*go*) _____ to graduate school.

5. Sarosh found out what was happening by (*listen*) _____ carefully to everything that was said.

6. Michelle works 16 hours a day in order (*earn*) _____ enough money (*take*) _____ care of her elderly parents and her three children.

7. No matter how wonderful a trip is, it's always good (*get*) _____ back home and (*sleep*) _____ in your own bed.

8. I keep (*forget*) _____ to call my friend Jae. I'd better write myself a note.

9. Exercise is good for you. Why don't you walk up the stairs instead of (*use*) _____ the elevator?

## EXERCISE 48 ▶ Check your knowledge. (Chapter 13 Review)
Correct the errors in the use of infinitives, gerunds, prepositions, and word order.

1. It is important getting an education.
   *to get*

2. I went to the bank for cashing a check.

3. Did you go to shopping yesterday?

4. I cut the rope by a knife.

5. I thanked my friend for drive me to the airport.

6. Is difficult to learn another language.

7. Timmy isn't enough old to get married.

8. Is easy this exercise to do.

9. Last night too tired no do my homework.

10. I've never gone to sailing, but I would like to.

11. Reading it is one of my hobbies.

12. The teenagers began to built a campfire to keep themselves warm.

13. Instead of settle down in one place, I'd like to travel around the world.

14. I enjoy to travel because you learn so much about other countries and cultures.

15. My grandmother likes to fishing.

16. Martina would like to has a big family.

# EXERCISE 49 ▸ Reading and grammar. (Chapter 13)

**Part I.** Read the passage.

> Do you know these words?
> - embarrassing
> - manufacture
> - shipping company
> - take a deep breath
> - ground floor
> - helplessly
> - grab
> - incident

### An Embarrassing Experience

Have you ever had an embarrassing experience? My Uncle Ernesto did while he was on a business trip in Norway.

Uncle Ernesto is a businessman from Buenos Aires, Argentina. He manufactures equipment for ships and needs to travel around the world to sell his products. Last year, he went to Norway to meet with a shipping company. While he was there, he found himself in an uncomfortable situation.

Uncle Ernesto was staying at a small hotel in Oslo. One morning, as he was getting ready to take a shower, he heard a knock at the door. He opened it, but no one was there. He stepped into the hallway. He still didn't see anyone, so he turned to go back to his room. Unfortunately, the door was locked. This was a big problem because he didn't have his key, and he was wearing only a towel.

Instead of standing in the hallway like this, he decided to get help at the front desk and started walking toward the elevator. He hoped to find an empty elevator, but the one that stopped had people in it. He took a deep breath and got in. The people in the elevator were surprised when they saw a man with a towel around him.

Uncle Ernesto thought about trying to explain his problem, but unfortunately he didn't know Norwegian. He knew a little English, so he said, "Door. Locked. No key." A businessman in the elevator nodded, but he wasn't smiling. Another man looked at Uncle Ernesto with a friendly smile.

The elevator seemed to move very slowly for Uncle Ernesto, but it finally reached the ground floor. He walked straight to the front desk and looked at the hotel manager helplessly. The hotel manager didn't have to understand any language to figure out the problem. He grabbed a key and led my uncle to the nearest elevator.

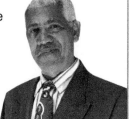

My uncle is still embarrassed about this incident. But he laughs a lot when he tells the story.

**Part II.** Check (✓) all the sentences that are grammatically correct.

1. a. _____ Uncle Ernesto went to Norway for a business meeting.
   b. _____ Uncle Ernesto went to Norway to have a business meeting.
   c. _____ Uncle Ernesto went to Norway for having a business meeting.

2. a. _____ Is necessary for him to travel in order to sell his products.
   b. _____ To sell his products, he needs to travel.
   c. _____ In order to sell his products, he needs to travel.

3. a. _____ Instead staying in the hall, he decided to get help.
   b. _____ Instead of staying in the hall, he decided to get help.
   c. _____ Instead to stay in the hall, he decided to get help.

4. a. _____ Uncle Ernesto thought about trying to explain his problem.
   b. _____ Uncle Ernesto considered about trying to explain his problem.
   c. _____ Uncle Ernesto decided not to explain his problem.

5. a. _____ It wasn't difficult for the hotel manager figuring out the problem.

   b. _____ It wasn't difficult for the hotel manager figure out the problem.

   c. _____ It wasn't difficult for the hotel manager to figure out the problem.

## EXERCISE 50 ▶ Reading and writing. (Chapter 13)

**Part I.** Read the passage.

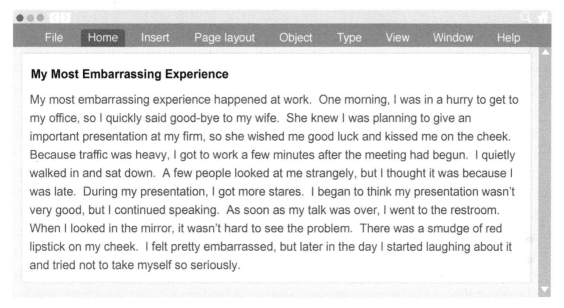

**My Most Embarrassing Experience**

My most embarrassing experience happened at work. One morning, I was in a hurry to get to my office, so I quickly said good-bye to my wife. She knew I was planning to give an important presentation at my firm, so she wished me good luck and kissed me on the cheek. Because traffic was heavy, I got to work a few minutes after the meeting had begun. I quietly walked in and sat down. A few people looked at me strangely, but I thought it was because I was late. During my presentation, I got more stares. I began to think my presentation wasn't very good, but I continued speaking. As soon as my talk was over, I went to the restroom. When I looked in the mirror, it wasn't hard to see the problem. There was a smudge of red lipstick on my cheek. I felt pretty embarrassed, but later in the day I started laughing about it and tried not to take myself so seriously.

**Part II.** Write a narrative paragraph about one of the most embarrassing experiences you have had in your life. Include some gerunds and infinitives in your writing.

> **WRITING TIP**
>
> A narrative paragraph tells a story or describes an event. It has a strong beginning, middle, and end. Follow these steps:
>
> 1. Set the scene with your topic sentence.
> 2. Tell what happened step by step. Time words/expressions help the reader follow your story. Note these examples in the above paragraph: *One morning, During my presentation, As soon as, When, later in the day.*
> 3. Finish with a strong concluding sentence.

**Part III.** Edit your writing. Check for the following:

1. ☐ use of some gerunds and infinitives
2. ☐ correct gerund forms
3. ☐ correct infinitive forms
4. ☐ use of some time words and expressions to help the reader follow the events
5. ☐ topic and concluding sentences
6. ☐ correct spelling (use a dictionary or spell-check)

---

▪▪▪▪▪ For digital resources, go to the Pearson Practice English app.

## PRETEST: What do I already know?

Write "C" if the sentences are correct and "I" if they are incorrect.

1. _____ I don't know how much this phone costs.  (Chart 14-1)

2. _____ Do you know whose is this seat?  (Chart 14-2)

3. _____ Dr. Mackey is wondering her patient will get better.  (Chart 14-3)

4. _____ Tommy dreamed a two-headed monster was chasing him.  (Chart 14-4)

5. _____ Is true that are you getting married?  (Chart 14-5)

6. _____ A:  Is Dorothy going to be 100 years old next week?  (Chart 14-6)

   B:  I think so.

7. _____ Professor Rico said, "Learning another language is hard work."  "It takes a long time."
   (Chart 14-7)

8. _____ Thomas said that he needed a ride to work.  (Chart 14-8)

9. _____ Emma said that she had studied Japanese in Tokyo.  (Chart 14-9)

10. _____ Jan told to us that she needed to go home early.  (Chart 14-10)

## EXERCISE 1 ▶ Warm-up.  (Chart 14-1)

Check (✓) all the grammatically correct sentences.

1. _____ How much does a smart watch cost?

2. _____ I don't know how much a smart watch costs.

3. _____ How much a smart watch costs?

4. _____ I don't know how much does a smart watch costs.

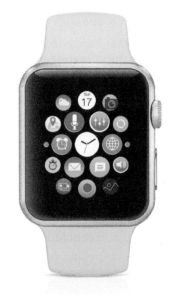

## 14-1 Noun Clauses: Introduction

| | |
|---|---|
| (a) S V O<br>I know *his address*.<br>(noun phrase) | Verbs are often followed by objects. The object is usually a noun phrase.*<br>In (a): *his address* is a noun phrase;<br>    *his address* is the object of the verb *know*. |
| (b) S V O<br>I know *where he lives*.<br>(noun clause) | Some verbs can be followed by noun clauses.*<br>In (b): *where he lives* is a noun clause;<br>    *where he lives* is the object of the verb *know*. |
| (c) S V O<br>           S V<br>I know *where he lives*. | A noun clause has its own subject and verb.<br>In (c): *he* is the subject of the noun clause;<br>    *lives* is the verb of the noun clause. |
| (d) I know *where my book is*.<br>(noun clause) | A noun clause can begin with a question word. (See Chart 14-2.) |
| (e) I don't know *if Ed is married*.<br>(noun clause) | A noun clause can begin with *if* or *whether*. (See Chart 14-3.) |
| (f) I know *that the world is round*.<br>(noun clause) | A noun clause can begin with *that*. (See Chart 14-4.) |

*A *phrase* is a group of related words. It does NOT contain a subject and a verb.
 A *clause* is a group of related words. It contains a subject and a verb.

### EXERCISE 2 ▸ Looking at grammar. (Chart 14-1)
Underline the noun clauses. One sentence has no noun clause.

**Former Neighbors**

1. Where are the Smiths living?
2. I don't know where the Smiths are living.
3. We don't know what city they moved to.
4. We know that they moved a month ago.
5. Are they coming back?
6. I don't know if they are coming back.

### EXERCISE 3 ▸ Warm-up: pairwork. (Chart 14-2)
Work with a partner. Ask and answer the questions. Make true statements.

1. PARTNER A: Where do I live?
   PARTNER B: I know/don't know where you live.

2. PARTNER B: Where does our teacher live?
   PARTNER A: I know/don't know where our teacher lives.

3. PARTNER B: In your last sentence, why is *does* missing?
   PARTNER A: I know/don't know why *does* is missing.

4. PARTNER A: In the same sentence, why does *lives* have an "s"?
   PARTNER B: I know/don't know why *lives* has an "s."

## 14-2 Noun Clauses That Begin with a Question Word

These question words can be used to introduce a noun clause: **when, where, why, how, who, (whom), what, which, whose**.

| Information Question | Noun Clause | Note in examples (a)–(f): |
|---|---|---|
| Where *does he live?* | (a) I don't know *where he lives*. | Usual question word order is NOT used in a noun clause. |
| When *did they leave?* | (b) Do you know *when they left?* | INCORRECT: *I know where does he live.*<br>CORRECT: I know where he lives. |
| What *did she say?* | (c) Please tell me *what she said*. | Note the question mark in (b), which includes a noun clause as part of the question. |
| Why *is Tom absent?* | (d) I wonder *why Tom is absent*. | |
| Who *is that boy?* | (e) Tell me *who that boy is*. | A noun or pronoun that follows main verb **be** in a question comes in front of **be** in a noun clause, as in (e) and (f). |
| Whose pen *is this?* | (f) Do you know *whose pen this is?* | |
| *Who is in the office?* | (g) I don't know *who is in the office*. | A prepositional phrase (e.g., *in the office*) does not come in front of **be** in a noun clause, as in (g) and (h). |
| *Whose keys are on the counter?* | (h) I wonder *whose keys are on the counter*. | |
| *Who came to class?* | (i) I don't know *who came to class*. | In (i) and (j): Question word order and noun clause word order are the same when the question word is used as a subject. |
| *What happened?* | (j) Tell me *what happened*. | |

In example (a): s = *he*, v = *lives*. In (b): s = *they*, v = *left*. In (c): s = *she*, v = *said*. In (d): s = *Tom*, v = *is*. In (e): v = *is*, s = *that boy*; noun clause s = *that boy*, v = *is*. In (f): v = *is*, s = *this*; noun clause s = *this*, v = *is*. In (g): s = *Who*, v = *is*; noun clause s = *who*, v = *is*. In (h): s = *Whose keys*, v = *are*; noun clause s = *whose keys*, v = *are*. In (i): s = *who*, v = *came*. In (j): s = *what*, v = *happened*.

## EXERCISE 4 ▶ Looking at grammar. (Charts 5-2 and 14-2)

**Part I.** If the sentence contains a noun clause, <u>underline</u> it and circle *noun clause*. If the question word introduces a question, circle *question*. Add final punctuation.

**Campus Questions**

1. Where is the library                                    noun clause     question
2. I'm not sure where the library is                       noun clause     question
3. What time does the bookstore open                       noun clause     question
4. Do you know what time the bookstore opens                noun clause     question
5. I wonder how we get tickets to the basketball game       noun clause     question
6. Do you know how we get tickets to the basketball game    noun clause     question

**Part II.** Compete the sentences with the given words. You may need to change the verb form. Add final punctuation.

1. *the bus / come*

    a. When ___does the bus come?___

    b. I don't know when ___the bus comes.___

2. *the bookstore / is*

    a. How far _____

    b. I don't know how far _____

3. *students / park their cars*

    a. Where _____

    b. Tell me where _____

4. *the gym / close early yesterday*

    a. Why did _____

    b. I'd like to know why _____

## EXERCISE 5 ▸ Looking at grammar. (Chart 14-2)
Choose the correct completions.

Questions Children Ask

1. Why _____ hot?
    a. is fire          b. fire is

2. I don't know why _____ hot.
    a. is fire          b. fire is

3. Do you know what _____ made of?
    a. the moon is      b. is the moon

4. Can you tell me why _____ blue?
    a. the sky is       b. is the sky

5. Can you explain where _____ from?
    a. does wind come   b. wind comes

6. Why _____ a tail?
    a. does a dog have  b. a dog has

7. I don't know why _____ a tail.
    a. does a dog have  b. a dog has

8. Do you know why _____?
    a. people die       b. do people die

9. How many bones _____?

    a. do I have           b. I have

10. Can you explain why _____ salt water?

    a. an ocean has     b. does an ocean have

## EXERCISE 6 ▸ Let's talk: pairwork. (Chart 14-2)

Work with a partner. Take turns asking questions. Begin with *Can you tell me*.

Questions to a Teacher

1. How do I pronounce this word? → *Can you tell me how I pronounce this word?*
2. What does this mean?
3. When will I get my grades?
4. What is our next assignment?
5. How soon is the next assignment due?
6. Why is this incorrect?
7. When is a good time to meet?
8. What day does the term end?
9. Why did I fail?
10. Who will teach this class next term?

## EXERCISE 7 ▸ Looking at grammar. (Chart 14-2)

Complete the responses with noun clauses.

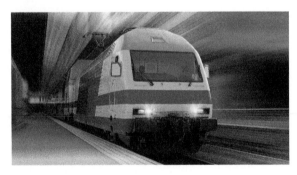

A Subway Ride

1. A: What is the next stop?

    B: I don't know *what the next stop is* .

2. A: How often does the train come?

    B: I don't know *how often the train comes* .

3. A: Where do you want to sit?

    B: I don't know _____.

4. A: Where do we get off?

    B: I'll ask _____.

5. A: Who's going to meet us?

   B: I'm not sure _____.

6. A: Whose phone is on the floor?

   B: I don't know _____.

7. A: What's that noise?

   B: I don't know _____.

8. A: Why are we stopping now?

   B: I have no idea _____.

9. A: Why is the alarm going off?

   B: I don't know _____.

10. A: What time is the last train?

    B: I'm not sure _____.

**EXERCISE 8 ▸ Let's talk: pairwork.** (Chart 14-2)
Work with a partner. Take turns asking questions. Begin with *Do you know*.

Questions at Home

1. Where is the phone?
2. Why is the front door open?
3. Who just called?
4. Whose socks are on the floor?
5. Why are all the lights on?
6. There's water all over the floor. What happened?
7. What did the plumber say about the broken pipe?
8. What is the repair going to cost?

**EXERCISE 9 ▸ Looking at grammar.** (Charts 5-2 and 14-2)
Complete the sentences with the correct form of the words in parentheses. There may be more than one answer for some.

Parents to Teens

1. A: Where (*you, go*) ____*did you go*____ last night?

   B: I thought Dad told you where (*we, go*) _____*we went*_____ last night.

2. A: It looks like you're getting ready to leave. Where (*you, go*) _____

   _____?

   B: I'm sorry. I didn't catch that.

   A: Oh, I was wondering where (*you, go*) _____

   _____.

3. A: Who (*you, text*) _____ right now?

   B: Why are you asking who (*I, text*) _____?

4. A: What time (*you, get*) _____ home last night?

   B: Who?

   A: You! I want to know what time (*you, get*) _____ home.

   B: Uh, kind of late.

5. A: Who (*you, meeting*) _____

   _____ after school tomorrow?

   B: I thought I told you who (*I, meet*) _____

   _____ after school.

6. A: When (*you, have*) _____ time to do your homework tomorrow?

   B: Pardon?

   A: I was wondering when (*you, have*) _____ time to do your homework.

7. A: What day (*your final exam, be*) _____

   _____?

   B: I'm not yet sure what day (*my final exam / be*) _____

   _____.

8. A: It looks like you were up all night. How much (*you, sleep*) _____?

   B: You want to know how much (*I, sleep*) _____?

   A: Yes, you look really tired.

## EXERCISE 10 ▶ Warm-up. (Chart 14-3)
Check (✓) all the grammatically correct sentences.

*Is Sam at work?*

1. _____ I don't know if Sam is at work.

2. _____ I don't know Sam is at work.

3. _____ I don't know if Sam is at work or not.

4. _____ I don't know whether Sam is at work.

| 14-3 Noun Clauses That Begin with *If* or *Whether* | | |
|---|---|---|
| **Yes/No Question** | **Noun Clause** | When a *yes/no* question is changed to a noun clause, *if* is usually used to introduce the clause.* |
| Is Eric at home? | (a) I don't know *if Eric is at home*. | |
| Does the bus stop here? | (b) Do you know *if the bus stops here*? | |
| Did Ava go to Bangkok? | (c) I wonder *if Ava went to Bangkok*. | |
| (d) I don't know *if Eric is at home or not*. | | When *if* introduces a noun clause, the expression ***or not*** sometimes comes at the end of the clause, as in (d). |
| (e) I don't know *whether Eric is at home (or not)*. | | In (e): ***whether*** has the same meaning as *if*. |

*See Chart 14-10 for the use of ***if*** with ***ask*** in reported speech.

## EXERCISE 11 ▸ Looking at grammar. (Chart 14-3)

Change the *yes/no* questions to noun clauses. Add final punctuation.

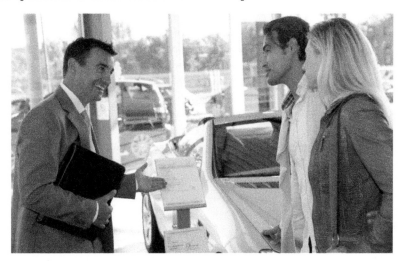

Buying a Car

1. *Yes/No* Question:    Is the price negotiable?

     Noun Clause:    Can you tell me __*if/whether the price is negotiable?*__

2. *Yes/No* Question:    Are online prices going to be better?

     Noun Clause:    I'd like to know _____

3. *Yes/No* Question:    Is there a warranty?

     Noun Clause:    Could you tell me _____

4. *Yes/No* Question:    Are other colors available?

     Noun Clause:    Could you check _____

5. *Yes/No* Question:    Is the car I want here?

     Noun Clause:    Do you know _____

6. *Yes/No* Question:    Has the car been in an accident?

     Noun Clause:    Can you check _____

7. *Yes/No* Question:    Do you take trade-ins?

     Noun Clause:    I'd like to know _____

8. *Yes/No* Question:    Does this car have a backup camera?

     Noun Clause:    Can you tell me _____

**EXERCISE 12 ▸ Looking at grammar.** (Chart 14-3)
Complete the noun clause in each conversation. Use *if* to introduce the
noun clause.

What was that?

1. A: Are you leaving?

   B: Sorry, I didn't catch that.

   A: I wanted to know __*if you are leaving*__.

2. A: Are you going to pick up the groceries?

   B: Pardon?

   A: I need to know _____ pick up the groceries.

3. A: Did you take my phone by accident?

   B: You had an accident?

   A: No! I want to know _____ my phone by accident.

4. A: Would you like to go to a movie tonight?

   B: Sorry – it's noisy in here. What was that?

   A: I'm wondering _____ to a movie tonight.

5. A: Are my car keys in the kitchen?

   B: Why are you asking me that? I have no idea _____

   in the kitchen.

   A: Someone woke up on the wrong side of the bed\*!

6. A: Is there gas in the car?

   B: What was that?

   A: I'm asking _____.

**EXERCISE 13 ▸ Let's talk: interview.** (Charts 14-2 and 14-3)
Interview your classmates. Begin your questions with **Do you know**. Answer with **I know** or
**I don't know**.

1. What does it cost to fly from London to Paris?
2. When was this building built?
3. How far is it from Vancouver, Canada, to Riyadh, Saudi Arabia?
4. Is Australia the smallest continent?
5. How many eyes does a bat have?
6. What is one of the longest words in English?
7. Does a chimpanzee have a good memory?

---

\**wake up on the wrong side of the bed* = wake up in a bad mood

8. How old is the Great Wall of China?
9. Do all birds fly?
10. Did birds come from dinosaurs?

**EXERCISE 14 ▸ Let's talk.** (Charts 14-2 and 14-3)
Work in small groups. Choose a famous movie star or celebrity. Make complete statements using noun clauses and the given words. Share some of your sentences with the class. See if anyone knows the information.

1. What do you wonder about him/her?
   a. where → *I wonder where she lives.*
   b. what
   c. if
   d. who
   e. how
   f. why

2. What do you want to ask him/her?
   a. who → *I want to ask him who his friends are.*
   b. when
   c. what
   d. whether
   e. why
   f. where

**EXERCISE 15 ▸ Let's talk: pairwork.** (Charts 14-2 and 14-3)
Work with a partner. Partner A asks the question. Partner B restates it with ***I'd like to know***.

At a Bank

| PARTNER A | PARTNER B |
|---|---|
| 1. What is the exchange rate? | 1. Can I apply for a credit card? |
| 2. Is there a fee for the ATM? | 2. What ID do you need? |
| 3. Are checks free? | 3. What is the late fee for a credit card payment? |
| 4. When will my debit card come? | 4. What is the minimum amount to open an account? |
| 5. What is the interest rate for a savings account? | 5. Is the account free? |
| | *Change roles.* |

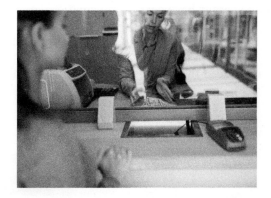

**EXERCISE 16 ▸ Warm-up.** (Chart 14-4)
Check (✓) all the grammatically correct sentences. Which checked sentences do you agree with?

1. _____ I think that noun clauses are hard.

2. _____ I think that this exercise is easy.

3. _____ I suppose that this chapter is useful.

4. _____ Is interesting this chapter I think.

## 14-4 Noun Clauses That Begin with *That*

| | |
|---|---|
| (a) $\overset{\text{S}}{\text{I}}\ \overset{\text{V}}{\text{think}}\ \overset{\text{O}}{\text{that Mr. Jones is a good teacher.}}$ <br> (b) I hope *that you can come to the game.* <br> (c) Mary realizes *that she should study harder.* <br> (d) I dreamed *that I was on the top of a mountain.* | A noun clause can be introduced by the word ***that***. <br><br> In (a): *that Mr. Jones is a good teacher* is a noun clause. It is the object of the verb ***think***. <br><br> *That*-clauses are frequently used as the objects of verbs that express mental activity. |
| (e) I think *that Mr. Jones is a good teacher.* <br> (f) I think Ø *Mr. Jones is a good teacher.* | The word ***that*** is often omitted, especially in speaking. Examples (e) and (f) have the same meaning. |

**Common Verbs Followed by *That*-clauses**

| | | | |
|---|---|---|---|
| agree that | dream that | know that | realize that |
| assume that | feel that | learn that | remember that |
| believe that | forget that | notice that | say that |
| decide that | guess that | predict that | suppose that |
| discover that | hear that | prove that | think that |
| doubt that | hope that | read that | understand that |

**EXERCISE 17 ▸ Grammar and speaking.** (Chart 14-4)
Add the word ***that*** to mark the beginning of a noun clause. Choose *yes* if you agree or *no* if you disagree. Then tell your partner your opinions by making true statements.

Social Media

1. I feel ^*that* people spend too much time on social media.     yes     no

2. I think social media is a good way for teens to communicate.     yes     no

3. I don't believe young children need to use social media.     yes     no

4. I think social media posts generally have correct information.     yes     no

5. Do you agree schools should teach kids how to use social media wisely?     yes     no

6. Do you think parents need to read their children's social media posts?     yes     no

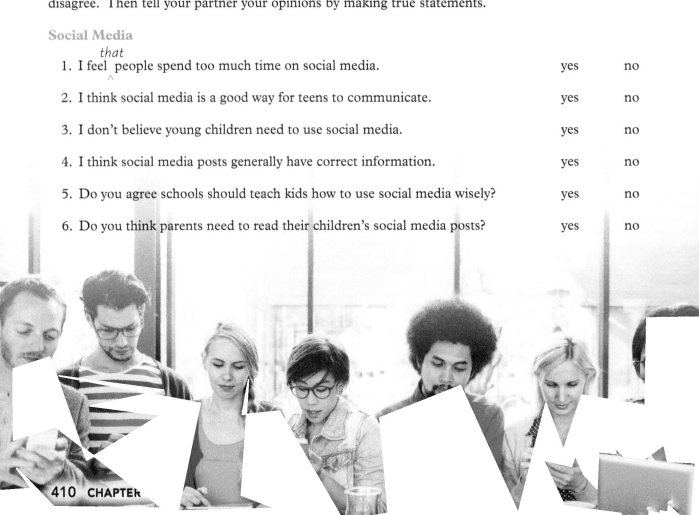

**EXERCISE 18 ▸ Let's talk: pairwork.** (Chart 14-4)
Work with a partner. Take turns asking and answering questions. Use *that*-clauses. Share some of your partner's answers with the class.

1. What have you noticed about English grammar?

2. What have you heard in the news recently?

3. What did you dream recently?

4. What do you believe about people?

5. What can scientists prove?

6. What can't scientists prove?

**EXERCISE 19 ▸ Warm-up.** (Chart 14-5)
Check (✓) the sentences that you agree with.

1. _____ I'm sure that vitamins give people more energy.

2. _____ It's true that vitamins help people live longer.

3. _____ It's a fact that vitamins help people look younger.

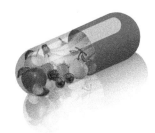

### 14-5 Other Uses of *That*-Clauses

| | |
|---|---|
| (a) I'm *sure that* the bus stops here. | *That*-clauses can follow certain expressions with **be** + *adjective* or **be** + *past participle*. |
| (b) I'm *glad that* you're feeling better today. | |
| (c) I'm *sorry that* I missed class yesterday. | The word ***that*** can be omitted with no change in meaning: |
| (d) I was *disappointed that* you couldn't come. | I'm sure *Ø* the bus stops here. |
| (e) *It is true that* the world is round. | Note two common expressions followed by *that*-clauses: |
| (f) *It is a fact that* the world is round. | It is true (that) ...<br>It is a fact (that) ... |

**Common Expressions Followed by *That*-clauses**

| | | | |
|---|---|---|---|
| be afraid that | be disappointed that | be sad that | be upset that |
| be angry that | be glad that | be shocked that | be worried that |
| be aware that | be happy that | be sorry that | |
| be certain that | be lucky that | be sure that | It is a fact that |
| be convinced that | be pleased that | be surprised that | It is true that |

**EXERCISE 20 ▸ Looking at grammar.** (Chart 14-5)
Add *that* where possible.

**At a Party**

1. A: Welcome. We're glad ^*that* you could come.

   B: Thank you. I'm happy I was able to make it.

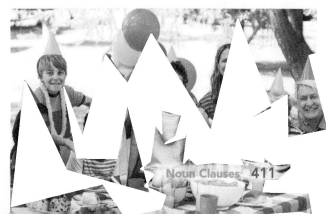

2. A: Thank you so much for your gift.

 B: I'm pleased you like it.

3. A: Are you surprised Paulo came but not Andrea?

 B: Yes! I'm certain she was invited.

4. A: Are you aware we are running out of food?

 B: No, we're not! I'm sure there's more in the kitchen.

 **EXERCISE 21 ▶ Let's talk.** (Charts 14-4 and 14-5)
**Part I.** Work in small groups. Look at the health treatments below.
Which ones do you know about? You may need to check your dictionary.

| | | |
|---|---|---|
| acupuncture | massage | naturopathy |
| hypnosis | meditation | yoga |

**Part II.** Complete the sentences with words in the box.
Use noun clauses. Discuss your sentences with other students.

1. I believe/think _____ is useful for _____ .

2. I am certain _____ .

3. I am not convinced _____ .

**EXERCISE 22 ▶ Listening and grammar.** (Charts 14-4 and 14-5)
Listen to each conversation and then complete the sentences. Answers may vary.

*Example:* You will hear: MAN:  I heard Jack is in jail. I can't believe it!
  WOMAN:  Neither can I! The police said he robbed a house.
    They must have the wrong person.
 You will say:  a. The man is shocked that <u>Jack is in jail</u>.
    b. The woman is sure that <u>the police have the wrong person</u>.

1. a. The woman thinks that ...        4. a. The man is happy that ...
 b. The man is glad that ...          b. The woman is pleased that ...

2. a. The mother is worried that ...    5. a. The woman is afraid* that ...
 b. Her son is sure that ...            b. The man is sure that ...

3. a. The man is surprised that ...
 b. The woman is disappointed that ...

---

*Sometimes **be afraid** expresses fear:
  *I don't want to go near that dog. I'm afraid that it will bite me.*
Sometimes **be afraid** expresses polite regret:
  *I'm afraid you have the wrong number.* = I'm sorry, but I think you have the wrong number.
  *I'm afraid I can't come to your party.* = I'm sorry, but I can't come to your party.

**EXERCISE 23 ▸ Reading and speaking.** (Charts 14-1 and 14-3 → 14-5)

**Part I.** Read the blog entry by co-author Stacy Hagen. Look at the sentences in green. Which ones have noun clauses? <u>Underline</u> the noun clauses.

Do you know these words?
- step back
- step forward
- rude
- back away
- signal
- distance
- acceptable
- imagine
- scene
- misunderstandings

# BlackBookBlog

## Personal Space

Sometimes a student stands really close to me during a conversation. I take a step back and the student steps forward. I take another step back, but the student moves forward again. What is happening? Is it rude when I step back? Do you think that I am being unfriendly?

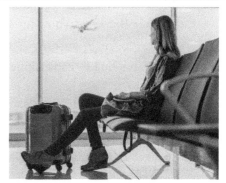

My behavior is actually about personal space. When two people are talking, and one person backs away, this is a signal. The person is uncomfortable with the distance between the two of them.

The acceptable distance can be different in different cultures. Imagine the following scene. You get into an elevator. There are two people already there, one in each corner. Think about where you will stand. If you are in the U.S. or Canada and stand close to one of them, that person will probably move away from you. Americans and Canadians feel uncomfortable when others get too close to them. They like to have some space around them.

Let's say you are on a subway. The car is empty except for you and a woman. A man enters and sits down next to the woman. How do you think the woman will feel? Is she going to be comfortable? The answer is most likely "no." This is generally very strange behavior. It's possible that the woman will even feel that she is in danger.

It is important that you understand personal space. You don't want misunderstandings to occur because of how close you stand or sit next to someone.

**Part II.** Work with a partner. Answer the following questions.

1. Were you aware of the information in this blog? What specifically? Did anything surprise you?

2. What feels normal for personal space in your culture? Show it by standing and talking to one another. If you are living in another country, practice standing acceptable distances from one another.

3. Look at the picture in the blog. Imagine a woman is coming into the waiting area. She understands personal space customs. Where will she sit? Or, where won't she sit?

4. When you meet a person for the first time, how do you greet him or her? What about a friend? Is there any kind of touching, e.g., shaking hands? How much distance is there?

5. What do you do if someone is standing or sitting too close to you?

## EXERCISE 24 ▶ Warm-up. (Chart 14-6)
Choose <u>all</u> the statements that are true for each conversation.

1. A: Did Jonathan remember to get food for dinner tonight?
   B: I think so.
   a. Speaker B thinks Jonathan got food for dinner.
   b. Speaker B is sure that Jonathan got food for dinner.
   c. Speaker B doesn't know for sure if Jonathan got food for dinner.

2. A: Is Jonathan going to cook dinner?
   B: I hope not.
   a. Speaker B says Jonathan is not going to cook dinner.
   b. Speaker B doesn't know if Jonathan is going to cook dinner.
   c. Speaker B doesn't want Jonathan to cook dinner.

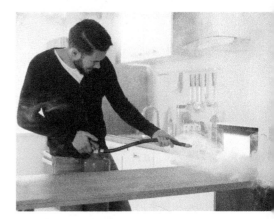

| 14-6 Substituting *So* for a *That*-Clause in Conversational Responses ||
|---|---|
| (a) A: Is Ana from Peru? <br> B: *I think so.* (*so = that Ana is from Peru*) | ***Think, believe,*** and ***hope*** are frequently followed by *so* in conversational English in response to a *yes/no* question. <br><br> ***So*** replaces a *that*-clause. <br> INCORRECT: *I think so that Ana is from Peru.* |
| (b) A: Does Olivia live in Montreal? <br> B: *I believe so.* (*so = that Olivia lives in Montreal*) | |
| (c) A: Did you pass the test? <br> B: *I hope so.* (*so = that I passed the test*) | |
| (d) A: Is Jack married? <br> B: *I don't think so. / I don't believe so.* | Negative usage of ***think so*** and ***believe so***: <br> *do not think so / do not believe so* |
| (e) A: Did you fail the test? <br> B: *I hope not.* | Negative usage of ***hope*** in conversational responses: <br> *hope not.* <br> In (e): ***I hope not*** = I hope I didn't fail the test. <br> INCORRECT: *I don't hope so.* |
| (f) A: Do you want to come with us? <br> B: Oh, I don't know. *I guess so.* | Other common conversational responses: <br>     *I guess so.*       *I guess not.* <br>     *I suppose so.*    *I suppose not.* <br> NOTE: In spoken English, ***suppose*** often sounds like "spoze." |

**EXERCISE 25 ▸ Looking at grammar.** (Chart 14-6)

Restate Speaker B's answers by using a *that*-clause.

**Weather Questions**

1. A: Is the sun going to come out?

   B: I hope so.

   → *I hope that the sun is going to come out.*

2. A: Will it rain tonight?

   B: I hope not.

3. A: Is a storm coming?

   B: I don't think so.

4. A: Do I hear hail on the roof?

   B: I think so.

5. A: Will the roads be icy tomorrow?

   B: I don't believe so.

**EXERCISE 26 ▸ Let's talk: pairwork.** (Chart 14-6)

Work with a partner. Take turns asking the questions. If you know the answer, use **Yes** or **No**. If you are not sure, use **I think so** or **I don't think so**.

*Example:*
SPEAKER A (*book open*):   Does this book have more than 500 pages?
SPEAKER B (*book closed*):  Yes, it does. / I don't think so. / etc.

| PARTNER A | PARTNER B |
|---|---|
| 1. Do you know how to spell my first name? | 1. Do you know how to spell my last name? |
| 2. Is your index finger bigger than your ring finger? | 2. Is your left foot bigger than your right foot? |
| 3. Is there a noun clause in this sentence? | 3. Do any English words begin with the letter "x"? |
| 4. Does the word *patient* have more than one meaning? | 4. Does the word *dozen* have more than one meaning? |
| 5. Do spiders have eyes? | 5. Do spiders have noses? |
| 6. Is there a fire extinguisher in this room? | 6. Is there a smoke alarm in this room? |
| 7. Is our teacher right-handed? | 7. Am I left-handed? |
| 8. Is this the last grammar exercise today? | 8. Does our teacher plan to give us homework today? |

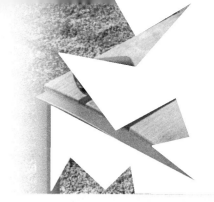

## EXERCISE 27 ▶ Warm-up. (Chart 14-7)

Circle the quotation marks and <u>underline</u> the punctuation inside each quotation. What are the differences in punctuation?

1. "Oh, no!" Vicki cried.

2. "Have you seen my wallet?" she asked.

3. "Maybe it's on the park bench that we were sitting on," I said.

---

## 14-7 Quoted Speech

Sometimes we want to quote a speaker's words — to write a speaker's exact words. Exact quotations are used in many kinds of writing, such as newspaper articles, stories, novels, and academic papers. When we quote a speaker's words, we use quotation marks.

| | |
|---|---|
| **(a)** SPEAKERS' EXACT WORDS<br>Jane: Cats are fun to watch.<br>Mike: Yes, I agree. They're graceful and playful. Do you have a cat? | **(b)** QUOTING THE SPEAKERS' WORDS<br>Jane said, "Cats are fun to watch."<br>Mike said, "Yes, I agree. They're graceful and playful. Do you have a cat?" |

**(c)** HOW TO WRITE QUOTATIONS

1. Add a comma after *said.*\* ──────────────▶ Jane said,
2. Add quotation marks.\*\* ──────────────▶ Jane said, "
3. Capitalize the first word of the quotation. ──────────▶ Jane said, "Cats
4. Write the quotation. Add a final period. ──────────▶ Jane said, "Cats are fun to watch.
5. Add quotation marks **after** the period. ──────────▶ Jane said, "Cats are fun to watch."

| | |
|---|---|
| **(d)** Mike said, "Yes, I agree. They're graceful and playful. Do you have a cat?"<br><br>**(e)** INCORRECT: *Mike said, "Yes, I agree." "They're graceful and playful." "Do you have a cat?"* | When there are two (or more) sentences in a quotation, put the quotation marks at the beginning and end of the whole quote, as in (d).<br><br>DO NOT put quotation marks around each sentence. As with a period, put the quotation marks after a question mark at the end of a quote. |
| **(f)** "Cats are fun to watch," Jane said.<br><br>**(g)** "Do you have a cat?" Mike asked. | In (f): Note that a comma (not a period) is used at the end of the QUOTED SENTENCE because **Jane said** comes after the quote.<br><br>In (g): Note that a question mark (not a comma) is used at the end of the QUOTED QUESTION. |

\*Other common verbs besides *say* that introduce quotations: *admit, announce, answer, ask, complain, explain, inquire, report, reply, shout, state, write.*

\*\*Quotation marks are called "inverted commas" in British English.

## EXERCISE 28 ▶ Looking at grammar. (Chart 14-7)

Make sentences in which you quote the speaker's exact words. Use **said** or **asked**. Punctuate carefully.

Problems

1. JULIANNA:   I forgot to pay my credit card bill.

   *Julianna said, "I forgot to pay my credit card bill."* OR

   *"I forgot to pay my credit card bill," Julianna said.*

2. RYAN:   I'm starving, and there's nothing in the fridge.

   _____

   _____

3. MEGAN:   I left my purse at home. I have no bus fare.

   _____

   _____

4. JON:   Did you miss the registration deadline too?

   _____

   _____

5. HAILEY:   We can't leave. I can't find the car keys.

   _____

   _____

## EXERCISE 29 ▶ Looking at grammar. (Chart 14-7)

A teacher recently had a conversation with Roberto. Punctuate their quoted speech.

(TEACHER)  You know sign language, don't you I asked Roberto.

(ROBERTO)  Yes, I do he replied both my grandparents are deaf.

(TEACHER)  I'm looking for someone who knows sign language. A deaf student is going
to visit our class next Monday I said. Could you interpret for her I asked.

(ROBERTO)  I'd be happy to he answered. Is she going to be a new student?

(TEACHER)  Possibly I said. She's interested in seeing what we do in our English classes.

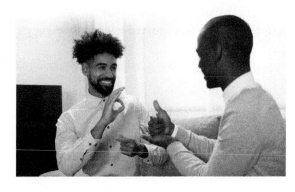

## EXERCISE 30 ▸ Warm-up. (Chart 14-8)

Circle the correct words.

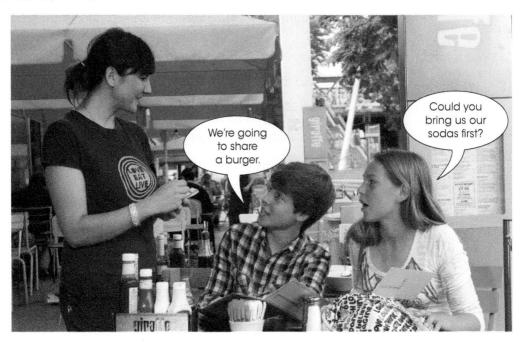

Noah and Jenna said that   we / they   were going to share a burger.

They wanted   our / their   sodas first.

| 14-8 | Quoted Speech vs. Reported Speech | |
| --- | --- | --- |
| QUOTED SPEECH<br><br>(a)  Ann said, *"I'm* hungry." <br>(b)  Tom said, *"I need my* pen." | QUOTED SPEECH = giving a speaker's exact words.  Quotation marks are used.* | |
| REPORTED SPEECH<br><br>(c)  Ann said (that) *she was* hungry. <br>(d)  Tom said (that) *he needed his* pen. | REPORTED SPEECH = giving the idea of a speaker's words.  Not all of the exact words are used; pronouns and verb forms may change.  Quotation marks are NOT used.*<br><br>***That*** is optional; it is more common in writing than in speaking. | |

*Quoted speech is also called *direct speech*.  Reported speech is also called *indirect speech*.

## EXERCISE 31 ▸ Looking at grammar. (Chart 14-8)

Change the pronouns from quoted speech to reported speech.

Voicemail

1. Maria said, "I will need help with my project."

   → Maria said that ___*she*___ would need help with ___*her*___ project.

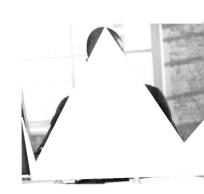

2. Ivan said, "I spoke with my client."

   → Ivan said that _____ spoke with _____ client.

3. Ellen said, "I am going to work from my home office the rest of the day."

   → Ellen said that _____ was going to work from _____ home office the rest of the day.

4. Rick said, "I'll meet you and Nora at your house after I finish my work at my house."

   → Rick said that _____ would meet _____ at _____ house after _____ finished _____ work at _____ house.

## EXERCISE 32 ▸ Warm-up. (Chart 14-9)

Read the conversation and look at the sentences that describe it. All are correct. What differences do you notice?

JENNY: What are you doing tomorrow?
ELLA: I'm going to take my parents out to dinner.

    a. Ella said she was going to take her parents out to dinner.
    b. Ella just said she is going to take her parents out to dinner.
    c. Last week Ella said she was going to take her parents out to dinner.
    d. Ella says she is going to take her parents out to dinner.

## 14-9 Verb Forms in Reported Speech

| | |
|---|---|
| (a) QUOTED:    Joe said, "I *feel* good."<br>(b) REPORTED: Joe said (that) he *felt* good.<br><br>(c) QUOTED:    Ken said, "I *am* happy."<br>(d) REPORTED: Ken said (that) he *was* happy. | In formal English, if the reporting verb (e.g., *said*) is in the past, the verb in the noun clause is often also in a past form, as in (b) and (d). |
|    — Ann said, "I am hungry."<br>(e)  — What did Ann just say? I didn't hear her.<br>   — She said (that) she *is* hungry.<br><br>(f)  — What did Ann say when she got home last night?<br>   — She said (that) she *was* hungry. | In informal English, often the verb in the noun clause is not changed to a past form, especially when words are reported *soon after* they are said, as in (e).<br><br>In *later reporting*, however, or in formal English, a past verb is commonly used, as in (f). |
| (g)  Ann **says** (that) she *is* hungry. | If the reporting verb is present tense (e.g., *says*), no change is made in the noun-clause verb. |

| QUOTED SPEECH | REPORTED SPEECH<br>(formal or later reporting) | REPORTED SPEECH<br>(informal or immediate reporting) |
|---|---|---|
| He said, "I *work* hard." | He said he *worked* hard. | He said he *works* hard. |
| He said, "I *am working* hard." | He said he *was working* hard. | He said he *is working* hard. |
| He said, "I *worked* hard." | He said he *had worked* hard. | He said he *worked* hard. |
| He said, "I *have worked* hard." | He said he *had worked* hard. | He said he *has worked* hard. |
| He said, "I *am going to work* hard." | He said he *was going to work* hard. | He said he *is going to work* hard. |
| He said, "I *will work* hard." | He said he *would work* hard. | He said he *will work* hard. |
| He said, "I *can work* hard." | He said he *could work* hard. | He said he *can work* hard. |

## EXERCISE 33 ▸ Looking at grammar. (Chart 14-9)

Complete the reported speech sentences. Use formal verb forms.

**Updates**

1. My advisor said, "I have updated your file."

   → My advisor said (that) she _____*had updated*_____ my file.

2. Kazu said, "I will finish soon."

   → Kazu said (that) he _____ soon.

3. I said, "Leo is meeting us for lunch instead of dinner."

   → I said (that) Leo _____ us for lunch instead of dinner.

4. Ben said, "I paid the overdue electric bill."

   → Ben said (that) he _____ the overdue electric bill.

5. Cyndi said, "I am going be out of town for two weeks."

   → Cyndi said (that) she _____ out of town for two weeks.

6. Ari said, "I can help my cousin move this weekend."

   → Ari said (that) he _____ his cousin move this weekend.

7. Tarik said to me, "I will take you to your appointment tomorrow."

   → Tarik said (that) he _____ me to my appointment tomorrow.

8. Kody said, "I don't feel like going out. I'm dealing with a broken heart."

   → Kody said (that) he _____ like going out. He _____

   with a broken heart.

## EXERCISE 34 ▸ Looking at grammar. (Charts 14-8 and 14-9)

Change the quoted speech to reported speech. Change the verb in quoted speech to a past form in reported speech if possible.

**Did I mention this?**

1. Jim said, "I'm getting a pet."
   → *Jim said (that) he was getting a pet.*
2. Kristina said, "I'm allergic to chocolate, nuts, and dairy."
3. Carla said, "I just came back from a trip with my family."
4. Ahmed said, "I have already picked up food for the party."
5. Kate said, "I called my doctor."
6. Mr. Rice said, "I'm going to go to Iceland for vacation."
7. Pedro said, "I will be at your house by noon."
8. Emma said, "I can't afford to buy a new car."
9. Olivia says, "I can't afford to buy a new car."
10. My dad said, "I want to print out some of my photos from my trip on your printer."

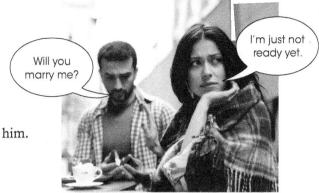

## EXERCISE 35 ▸ Warm-up. (Chart 14-10)
Choose all the grammatically correct sentences.

1. a. David asked Elena if she would marry him.
   b. David asked Elena would she marry him.
   c. David wanted to know if Elena would marry him.

2. a. Elena said she wasn't ready yet.
   b. Elena told she wasn't ready yet.
   c. Elena told David she wasn't ready yet.

| 14-10 Common Reporting Verbs: *Tell, Ask, Answer/Reply* | |
|---|---|
| (a) Kay *said* that* she was hungry.<br>(b) Kay *told me* that she was hungry.<br>(c) Kay *told Tom* that she was hungry.<br><br>INCORRECT: *Kay told that she was hungry.*<br>INCORRECT: *Kay told to me that she was hungry.*<br>INCORRECT: *Kay said me that she was hungry.* | A main verb that introduces reported speech is called a "reporting verb." **Say** is the most common reporting verb** and is usually followed immediately by a noun clause, as in (a).<br><br>**Tell** is also commonly used. Note that **told** is followed by **me** in (b) and by **Tom** in (c).<br><br>**Tell** needs to be followed immediately by a (pro)noun object and then by a noun clause. |
| (d) QUOTED: Ken asked me, "Are you tired?"<br>REPORTED: Ken *asked (me) if* I was tired. | **Asked** is used to report questions. |
| (e) Ken *wanted to know if* I was tired.<br>Ken *wondered if* I was tired.<br>Ken *inquired whether or not* I was tired. | Questions are also reported by using **want to know**, **wonder**, and **inquire**. |
| (f) QUOTED: I said (to Kay), "I am not tired."<br>REPORTED: I *answered / replied* that I wasn't tired. | The verbs **answer** and **reply** are often used to report replies. |

\**That* is optional. See Chart 14-8.

\*\*Other common reporting verbs: *Kay **announced** / **commented** / **complained** / **explained** / **remarked** / **stated** that she was hungry.*

## EXERCISE 36 ▸ Looking at grammar. (Chart 14-10)
Complete the sentences with **said, told,** or **asked.**

*By the way,*

1. Karen ___told___ me that she would be here at one o'clock.

2. Jamal ___said___ that he was going to get here around two.

3. Sophia ___asked___ me what time we would arrive.

4. William _____ that you had a message.

5. William _____ me that someone had called you around ten-thirty.

6. I _____ William if he knew the caller's name.

7. Alice called. I _____ her that I would help her move into her new apartment next week. She _____ that she would welcome the help. She _____ me if I had a truck or knew anyone who had a truck. I _____ her Dan had a truck. She _____ she would call him.

8. My uncle in Toronto called and _____ that he was organizing a surprise party for my aunt's 60th birthday. He _____ me if we could come to Toronto for the party. I _____ him that we would be happy to come. I _____ when it was. He _____ it was the last weekend in August.

**EXERCISE 37** ▸ **Let's talk: pairwork.** (Charts 14-2, 14-3, and 14-10)
Work with a partner. Write down five questions to ask your partner about his/her life or opinions. Note your partner's answers. Share some of the information with the class. Include both the question and the response. Use either formal or informal verb forms.*

*Examples:*
PARTNER A's question:   Where were you born?
PARTNER B's response:   In Nepal.
PARTNER A's report:     I asked him where he was born. He told me he was born in Nepal.

PARTNER B's question:   Who do you admire most in the world?
PARTNER A's response:   I admire my parents.
PARTNER B's report:     I asked him who he admires most in the world. He said he admires his parents the most.

**EXERCISE 38** ▸ **Looking at grammar.** (Charts 14-8 → 14-10)
Complete the paragraph based on what the people in the picture are saying. Use the formal sequence of tenses.

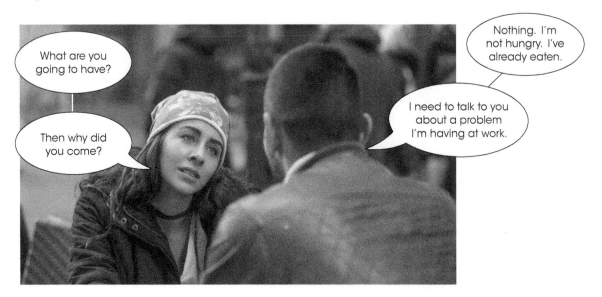

---

*In everyday spoken English, native speakers sometimes change formal/later noun-clause verbs to past forms, and sometimes they don't. In an informal reporting situation, either informal/immediate reporting or reporting tenses are appropriate.

One day Katya and Pavel were at a restaurant. Katya picked up her menu and looked at it. Pavel left his menu on the table. Katya asked Pavel _____what he was going to have_____ . He said

_____ anything because he
                                    2

_____ . He _____ already. Katya was
            3                               4

surprised. She asked him why _____ . He told her
                                              5

_____ about a problem _____
                        6                                                    7

at work.

## EXERCISE 39 ▶ Looking at grammar. (Charts 14-8 → 14-10)

Change the reported speech to quoted speech. Begin a new paragraph each time the speaker changes. Pay special attention to pronouns, verb forms, and word order. Answers may vary.

*Example:*

REPORTED SPEECH: This morning my mother asked me if I had gotten enough sleep last night. I told her that I was fine. I explained that I didn't need a lot of sleep. She told me that I needed to take better care of myself.

QUOTED SPEECH:    *This morning my mother asked, "Did you get enough sleep last night?"*

*"I'm fine," I replied. "I don't need a lot of sleep."*

*She said, "You need to take better care of yourself."*

1. In the middle of class yesterday, my friend tapped me on the shoulder and asked me what I was doing after class. I told her that I would tell her later.

   _____

   _____

   _____

2. When I was putting on my coat, Robert asked me where I was going. I told him that I had a date with Anna. He wanted to know what we were going to do. I told him that we were going to a movie.

   _____

   _____

   _____

   _____

3. This afternoon, a friend called and asked me if I had time to talk. She was thinking about taking a new job in another city. I said that I was at work, and I wasn't free to take a personal call. I asked if she could talk this evening, after dinner.

   _____

   _____

   _____

**EXERCISE 40 ▶ Listening.** (Charts 14-8 → 14-10)

Listen to Roger's report of his phone conversation with Angela. Then listen again and write the missing words.

Angela called and _____1_____ me where Bill _____2_____.

I _____3_____ her he _____4_____ in the lunchroom. She

_____5_____ when he _____6_____ back. I _____7_____

he _____8_____ back around 2:00. I _____9_____ her if I

_____10_____ something for her.

She _____11_____ that Bill had the information she _____12_____,

and only he _____13_____ her. I _____14_____ her that I

_____15_____ him a message. She thanked me and hung up.

**EXERCISE 41 ▶ Reading and speaking.** (Chapter 14 Review)

**Part I.** Read the passage.

# THE LAST LECTURE

Do you know these words?
- lecture series
- wisdom
- opportunity
- cancer
- uplifting
- achieving
- inspiring
- apology
- tend to
- key question

In 2007, a 47-year-old computer science professor from Carnegie Mellon University was invited to give a lecture at his university. His name was Randy Pausch, and the lecture series was called "The Last Lecture." Pausch was asked to think about what wisdom he would give to people if he knew it was his last opportunity to do so. In Pausch's case, it really was his last lecture because he had cancer and wasn't expected to survive. Pausch gave an uplifting lecture called "Really Achieving Your Childhood Dreams." The lecture was recorded and put on the internet. A reporter for the *Wall Street Journal* was also there and wrote about it. Soon millions of people around the world heard about Pausch's inspiring talk.

Here are some quotes from Randy Pausch:

*To the general public:*

"Proper apologies have three parts: (1) What I did was wrong. (2) I'm sorry that I hurt you. (3) How do I make it better? It's the third part that people tend to forget."

"If I could only give three words of advice, they would be 'tell the truth.' If I got three more words, I'd add 'all the time.' "

"The key question to keep asking is, 'Are you spending your time on the right things?' Because time is all you have."

"We cannot change the cards we are dealt, just how we play the hand."

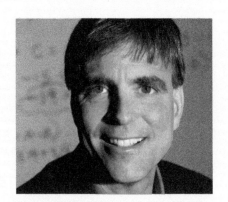

To his students: "Whether you think you can or can't, you're right."

To his children: "Don't try to figure out what I wanted you to become. I want you to become what you want to become."

Sadly, in 2008, Randy Pausch died. Before his death he was able to put down his thoughts in a book, appropriately called *The Last Lecture*.

**Part II.** Work in small groups. Explain the meaning of each quotation in Part I. Then, individually, choose one of the quotes to agree or disagree with. Use some of the phrases in the box and support your statement with reasons.

I agree / disagree that
I believe / don't believe that
I think / don't think that
It's true that

## EXERCISE 42 ▶ Check your knowledge. (Chapter 14 Review)
Correct the errors.

1. My friend knows where do I live.

2. I don't know what is your email address?

3. I think so that Mr. Lee is out of town.

4. Can you tell me that where Victor is living now?

5. I asked my uncle what kind of movies does he like.

6. I think, that my English has improved a lot.

7. Is true that people are basically the same everywhere in the world.

8. A man came to my door last week. I didn't know who is he.

9. I want to know does Pedro have a laptop computer.

10. Sam and I talked about his classes. He told that he don't like his algebra class.

11. A woman came into the room and ask me Where is your brother?

12. I felt very relieved when the doctor said, you will be fine. It's nothing serious.

13. My mother asked me that: "When you will be home?

**EXERCISE 43 ▸ Reading, grammar, and writing. (Chapter 14)**
**Part I.** Read the story. Add quotation marks and other necessary punctuation to the sentences in green. You may need to capitalize some letters.

Do you know these words?
- nest
- the rest
- hatch
- feathers
- clumsy
- slender
- wander
- bed of reeds
- plenty of
- reflection

## The Ugly Duckling

Once upon a time, there was a mother duck. She lived on a farm and spent her days sitting on her nest of eggs. One morning, the eggs began to move, and out came six little ducklings. But there was one egg that was bigger than the rest, and it didn't hatch. The mother didn't remember this egg. I thought I had only six, but maybe I counted incorrectly she said.

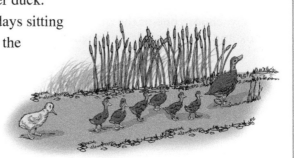

a mother duck and her ducklings

A short time later, the seventh egg hatched. But this duckling had gray feathers, not brown like his brothers, and was quite ugly. His mother thought, maybe this duck isn't one of mine. He grew faster than his brothers and ate more food. He was very clumsy, and none of the other animals wanted to play with him. Much of the time he was alone.

He felt unloved by everyone, and he decided to run away from the farm. He asked other animals on the way, do you know of any ducklings that look like me? But they just laughed and said you are the ugliest duck we have ever seen. One day, the duckling looked up and saw a group of beautiful birds overhead. They were white, with long, slender necks and large wings. I want to look just like them, the duckling thought.

He wandered alone most of the winter and finally found a comfortable bed of reeds in a pond. He thought to himself, no one wants me. I'll just hide here for the rest of my life. There was plenty of food there, and although he was lonely, he felt a little happier.

By springtime, the duck was quite large. One morning, he saw his reflection in the water. He didn't even recognize himself. A group of swans that was coming back from the south saw him and flew down to the pond. Where have you been? they cried. You're a swan like us. As they began to swim across the pond, a child saw them and exclaimed, look at the youngest swan. He's the most beautiful of all. The swan was filled with happiness, and he lived happily ever after.

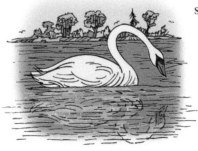

a swan

**Part II.** Work in small groups and answer this question: What lessons does this story teach? Share your answers with the class.

**Part III.** Write a story that includes quoted speech. Tell the actions or events of your story using verbs in a past tense.

1. Write a fable from your country in which animals speak. (A fable is a traditional story that teaches a lesson about life.) OR Write a story that you learned when you were young.

2. Take five minutes to tell a student your story. Then tell it to another student in four minutes. Finally, take three minutes to tell your story to a third student. The last time you speak should feel more comfortable and easier than the first time.

---

### WRITING TIP

The use of quoted speech can make a story feel more real or immediate to the reader. When you use quotes, it is a good idea to vary the style. *Say* is a common verb for introducing quoted speech, but, as you can see from this story, there are other verbs you can use. You can also vary the position of the verbs used with quoted speech: they can go at the beginning, in the middle, or at the end of a quotation.

Note the different verbs the writer used to introduce quotations in "The Ugly Duckling" and where they are placed. In general, the verb tense used in quoted speech is either in the present or present perfect. Of course, there are exceptions, such as the first quote in the story, which uses the simple past.

---

**Part IV.** Edit your writing. Check for the following:

1. ☐ use of some quoted speech
2. ☐ correct punctuation with quotation marks
3. ☐ correct capitalization with quotation marks
4. ☐ in general, use of the present or present perfect tense in quoted speech
5. ☐ in general, use of a past tense to tell the story
6. ☐ correct spelling (use a dictionary or spell-check)

---

▪▪▪▪▪ For digital resources, go to the Pearson Practice English app.

# Appendix

## Supplementary Grammar Charts

## UNIT A

### A-1 The Principal Parts of a Verb

#### Regular Verbs

| SIMPLE FORM | SIMPLE PAST | PAST PARTICIPLE | PRESENT PARTICIPLE |
|---|---|---|---|
| call | called | called | calling |
| clean | cleaned | cleaned | cleaning |
| plan | planned | planned | planning |
| play | played | played | playing |
| try | tried | tried | trying |

#### Irregular Verbs

| SIMPLE FORM | SIMPLE PAST | PAST PARTICIPLE | PRESENT PARTICIPLE |
|---|---|---|---|
| eat | ate | eaten | eating |
| break | broke | broken | breaking |
| come | came | come | coming |
| sing | sang | sung | singing |
| put | put | put | putting |

#### Principal Parts of a Verb

| (1) THE SIMPLE FORM | English verbs have four principal forms, or "parts." *The simple form* is the form that is found in a dictionary. It is the base form with no endings on it (no final *-s*, *-ed*, or *-ing*). |
|---|---|
| (2) THE SIMPLE PAST | *The simple past* ends in *-ed* for regular verbs. Most verbs are regular, but many common verbs have irregular past forms. |
| (3) THE PAST PARTICIPLE | *The past participle* also ends in *-ed* for regular verbs. Other verbs have irregular past participles. Past participles are used with the perfect tenses (Chapter 4) and the passive (Chapter 10). |
| (4) THE PRESENT PARTICIPLE | *The present participle* ends in *-ing* (for both regular and irregular verbs). It is used in progressive tenses (e.g., the present progressive and the past progressive). |

The woman *is calling* for help again. Her car *broke* down in the snow. She *called* for a tow truck an hour ago, but no one *has come* yet.

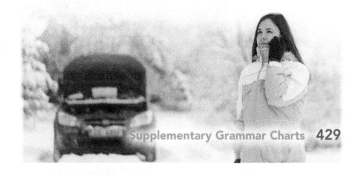

| SIMPLE FORM | SIMPLE PAST | PAST PARTICIPLE | SIMPLE FORM | SIMPLE PAST | PAST PARTICIPLE |
|---|---|---|---|---|---|
| be | was, were | been | lend | lent | lent |
| beat | beat | beaten | let | let | let |
| become | became | become | lie | lay | lain |
| begin | began | begun | light | lit/lighted | lit/lighted |
| bend | bent | bent | lose | lost | lost |
| bite | bit | bitten | make | made | made |
| blow | blew | blown | mean | meant | meant |
| break | broke | broken | meet | met | met |
| bring | brought | brought | pay | paid | paid |
| build | built | built | put | put | put |
| burn | burned/burnt | burned/burnt | quit | quit | quit |
| buy | bought | bought | read | read | read |
| catch | caught | caught | ride | rode | ridden |
| choose | chose | chosen | ring | rang | rung |
| come | came | come | rise | rose | risen |
| cost | cost | cost | run | ran | run |
| cut | cut | cut | say | said | said |
| dig | dug | dug | see | saw | seen |
| do | did | done | sell | sold | sold |
| draw | drew | drawn | send | sent | sent |
| dream | dreamed/dreamt | dreamed/dreamt | set | set | set |
| drink | drank | drunk | shake | shook | shaken |
| drive | drove | driven | shoot | shot | shot |
| eat | ate | eaten | shut | shut | shut |
| fall | fell | fallen | sing | sang | sung |
| feed | fed | fed | sink | sank | sunk |
| feel | felt | felt | sit | sat | sat |
| fight | fought | fought | sleep | slept | slept |
| find | found | found | slide | slid | slid |
| fit | fit | fit | speak | spoke | spoken |
| fly | flew | flown | spend | spent | spent |
| forget | forgot | forgotten | spread | spread | spread |
| forgive | forgave | forgiven | stand | stood | stood |
| freeze | froze | frozen | steal | stole | stolen |
| get | got | got/gotten | stick | stuck | stuck |
| give | gave | given | swim | swam | swum |
| go | went | gone | take | took | taken |
| grow | grew | grown | teach | taught | taught |
| hang | hung | hung | tear | tore | torn |
| have | had | had | tell | told | told |
| hear | heard | heard | think | thought | thought |
| hide | hid | hidden | throw | threw | thrown |
| hit | hit | hit | understand | understood | understood |
| hold | held | held | upset | upset | upset |
| hurt | hurt | hurt | wake | woke/waked | woken/waked |
| keep | kept | kept | wear | wore | worn |
| know | knew | known | win | won | won |
| leave | left | left | write | wrote | written |

## A-3 The Present Perfect vs. The Past Perfect

| PRESENT PERFECT | (a) I am not hungry now. I *have* already *eaten*. | The PRESENT PERFECT expresses an activity that *occurred before now*, at *an unspecified time in the past,* as in (a). |
|---|---|---|
| PAST PERFECT | (b) I was not hungry at 1:00 P.M. I *had* already *eaten*. | The PAST PERFECT expresses an activity that *occurred before **another** time in the past*.<br><br>In (b): I ate at noon. I was not hungry at 1:00 P.M. because I had already eaten before 1:00 P.M. |

## A-4 The Past Progressive vs. The Past Perfect

| PAST PROGRESSIVE | (a) I *was eating* when Bob came. | The PAST PROGRESSIVE expresses an activity that was *in progress at a particular time in the past*.<br><br>In (a): I began to eat at noon. Bob came at 12:10. My meal was in progress when Bob came. |
|---|---|---|
| PAST PERFECT | (b) I *had eaten* when Bob came. | The PAST PERFECT expresses an activity that was *completed before a particular time in the past*.<br><br>In (b): I finished eating at noon. Bob came at 1:00 P.M. My meal was completed before Bob came. |

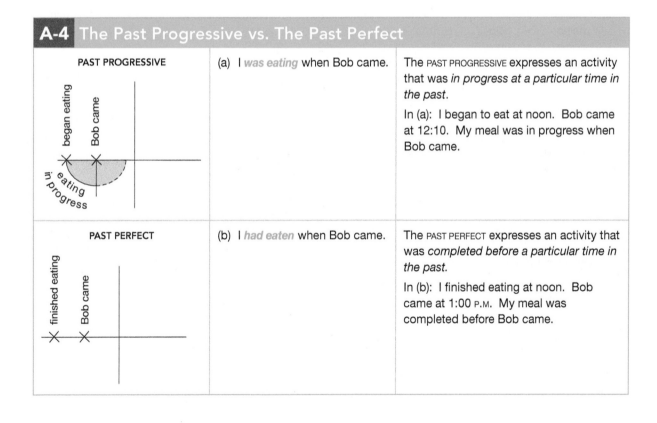

## A-5   Regular Verbs: Pronunciation of -ed Endings

| | | |
|---|---|---|
| (a) | talked = talk/t/<br>stopped = stop/t/<br>missed = miss/t/<br>watched = watch/t/<br>washed = wash/t/ | Final **-ed** is pronounced /t/ after voiceless sounds.<br>You make a voiceless sound by pushing air through your mouth.<br>No sound comes from your throat.<br>Examples of voiceless sounds: /k/, /p/, /s/, /ch/, /sh/. |
| (b) | called = call/d/<br>rained = rain/d/<br>lived = live/d/<br>robbed = rob/d/<br>stayed = stay/d/ | Final **-ed** is pronounced /d/ after voiced sounds.<br>You make a voiced sound from your throat. Your voice box vibrates.<br>Examples of voiced sounds: /l/, /n/, /v/, /b/, and all vowel sounds. |
| (c) | waited = wait/əd/<br>needed = need/əd/ | Final **-ed** is pronounced /əd/* after "t" and "d" sounds.<br>In (c): /əd/ adds a syllable to a word. |

*/əd/ is pronounced "ud."

## A-6   Pronunciation of Final -s/-es for Verbs and Nouns

Final **-s/-es** *on verbs and nouns* has three different pronunciations: /s/, /z/, and /əz/.

| | | |
|---|---|---|
| (a) | meets = meet/s/<br>helps = help/s/<br>books = book/s/ | Final **-s** is pronounced /s/ after voiceless sounds. In (a): /s/ is the sound of "s" in *bus*.<br>Examples of voiceless sounds: /t/, /p/, /k/. |
| (b) | needs = need/z/<br>wear = wear/z/<br>calls = call/z/<br>views = view/z/ | Final **-s** is pronounced /z/ after voiced sounds. In (b): /z/ is the sound of "z" in *buzz*.<br>Examples of voiced sounds: /d/, /r/, /l/, /m/, /b/, and all vowel sounds. |
| (c) | wishes = wish/əz/<br>watches = watch/əz/<br>passes = pass/əz/<br>sizes = size/əz/<br>pages = page/əz/<br>judges = judge/əz/ | Final **-s/-es** is pronounced /əz/* after *-sh, -ch, -s, -z, -ge/-dge* sounds.<br>In (c): /əz/ adds a syllable to a word. |

*/əz/ is pronounced "uz."

| SUBJECT PRONOUNS | OBJECT PRONOUNS | POSSESSIVE PRONOUNS | POSSESSIVE ADJECTIVES |
|---|---|---|---|
| I | me | mine | **my** name(s) |
| you | you | yours | **your** name(s) |
| she | her | hers | **her** name(s) |
| he | him | his | **his** name(s) |
| it | it | its | **its** name(s) |
| we | us | ours | **our** name(s) |
| you | you | yours | **your** name(s) |
| they | them | theirs | **their** name(s) |

| | |
|---|---|
| (a) *We* saw an accident. <br> (b) Sonya saw *it* too. <br> (c) I have my pen. Ella has *hers*. <br> (d) *Her* pen is blue. | Personal pronouns are used as: <br> • subjects, as in (a); <br> • objects, as in (b); OR <br> • to show possession, as in (c) <br> Possessive adjectives also show possession, as in (d). |
| (e) I have a *book*. *It* is on my desk. <br> (f) I have some *books*. *They* are on my desk. | Use a singular pronoun to refer to a singular noun. In (e): *book* and *it* are both singular. <br> Use a plural pronoun to refer to a plural noun. In (f): *books* and *they* are both plural. |
| (g) *It's* sunny today. <br> (h) I'm studying about India. I'm interested in *its* history. <br> INCORRECT: *I'm interested in it's history.* | COMPARE: In (g): **it's** = *it is* <br> In (h): **its** is a possessive adjective: <br>      *its history* = *India's history* <br> A possessive adjective has NO apostrophe. |

| (Question Word) | Helping Verb | Subject | Main Verb | (Rest of Sentence) | |
|---|---|---|---|---|---|
| (a) | *Does* | *Leo* | *live* | in Montreal? | |
| (b) Where | *does* | *Leo* | *live*? | | |
| (c) | *Is* | *Sara* | *studying* | at the library? | |
| (d) Where | *is* | *Sara* | *studying*? | | |
| (e) | *Will* | *you* | *help* | me? | |
| (f) When | *will* | *you* | *help* | me? | |
| (g) | *Did* | *they* | *see* | Mario? | |
| (h) Who(m) | *did* | *they* | *see*? | | |
| (i) | *Is* | *Olaf* | | at home? | |
| (j) Where | *is* | *Olaf*? | | | |
| (k) | | *Who* | *came*? | | When the question word (e.g., **who** or **what**) is the subject of the sentence, **do** or **does** is never used. |
| (l) | | *What* | *happened*? | | |

# UNIT B: Phrasal Verbs

NOTE: See the *Fundamentals of English Grammar Workbook* appendix for practice exercises for phrasal verbs.

## B-1 Phrasal Verbs

| | |
|---|---|
| (a) We *put off* our trip. We'll go next month instead of this month. (*put off = postpone*) | In (a): **put off** = a phrasal verb |
| | A PHRASAL VERB = a verb and a particle that together have a special meaning. For example, *put off* means "postpone." |
| (b) Jimmy, *put on* your coat before you go outdoors. (*put on  =  place clothes on one's body*) | |
| (c) Someone left the scissors on the table. They didn't belong there. I *put* them *away*. (*put away  =  put something in its usual or proper place*) | A PARTICLE = a "small word" (e.g., *off, on, away, back*) that is used in a phrasal verb. |
| (d) After I used the dictionary, I *put* it *back* on the shelf. (*put back  =  return something to its original place*) | Note that the phrasal verbs with **put** in (a), (b), (c), and (d) all have different meanings. |

### Separable

| | |
|---|---|
| (e) We *put off our trip*. = (VERB + **particle** + NOUN) | Some phrasal verbs are **separable**: A NOUN OBJECT can either |
| (f) We *put our trip off*. = (VERB + NOUN + **particle**) | (1) follow the particle, as in (e), OR<br>(2) come between (separate) the verb and the particle, as in (f). |
| (g) We *put it off*.        = (VERB + PRONOUN + **particle**) | If a phrasal verb is separable, a PRONOUN OBJECT comes between the verb and the particle, as in (g). |
| | *INCORRECT: We put off it.* |

### Nonseparable

| | |
|---|---|
| (h) I *ran into Bob*. = (VERB + **particle** + NOUN) | If a phrasal verb is **nonseparable**, a NOUN or PRONOUN always follows (never precedes) the particle, as in (h) and (i). |
| (i) I *ran into him*. = (VERB + **particle** + PRONOUN) | *INCORRECT: I ran Bob into.*<br>*INCORRECT: I ran him into.* |

### Phrasal Verbs: Intransitive

| | |
|---|---|
| (j) The machine *broke down*. | Some phrasal verbs are intransitive; i.e., they are not followed by an object. |
| (k) Please *come in*. | |
| (l) Mr. Lim *passed away*. | |

### Three-Word Phrasal Verbs

| | |
|---|---|
| (m) Last night some friends *dropped in*. | Some two-word verbs (e.g., *drop in*) can become three-word verbs (e.g., *drop in on*). |
| | In (m): **drop in** is not followed by an object. It is an intransitive phrasal verb (i.e., it is not followed by an object). |
| (n) Let's *drop in on* Alice this afternoon. | In (n): **drop in on** is a three-word phrasal verb. Three-word phrasal verbs are transitive (they are followed by objects). |
| (o) We *dropped in on her* last week. | In (o): Three-word phrasal verbs are nonseparable (the noun or pronoun follows the phrasal verb). |

A  **ask out** = ask (someone) to go on a date

B  **blow out** = extinguish (a match, a candle)
   **break down** = stop functioning properly
   **break out** = happen suddenly
   **break up** = separate, end a relationship
   **bring back** = return
   **bring up** = (1) raise (children)
               (2) mention, start to talk about

C  **call back** = return a telephone call
   **call off** = cancel
   **call on** = ask (someone) to speak in class
   **call up** = make a telephone call
   **cheer up** = make happier
   **clean up** = make neat and clean
   **come along (with)** = accompany
   **come from** = originate
   **come in** = enter a room or building
   **come over (to)** = visit the speaker's place
   **cross out** = draw a line through
   **cut out (of)** = remove with scissors or knife

D  **dress up** = put on nice clothes
   **drop in (on)** = visit without calling first or
                   without an invitation
   **drop out (of)** = stop attending (school)

E  **eat out** = eat at a restaurant

F  **fall down** = fall to the ground
   **figure out** = find the solution to a problem
   **fill in** = complete by writing in a blank space
   **fill out** = write information on a form
   **fill up** = fill completely with gas, water, coffee,
               etc.
   **find out (about)** = discover information
   **fool around (with)** = have fun while wasting
                         time

G  **get on** = enter a bus/an airplane/a train/a
              subway
   **get out of** = leave a car, a taxi

**get over** = recover from an illness or a shock
**get together (with)** = join, meet
**get through (with)** = finish
**get up** = get out of bed in the morning
**give away** = donate, get rid of by giving
**give back** = return (something) to (someone)
**give up** = quit doing (something) or quit trying
**go on** = continue
**go back (to)** = return to a place
**go out** = not stay home
**go over (to)** = (1) approach
                 (2) visit another's home
**grow up (in)** = become an adult

H  **hand in** = give homework, test papers, etc., to a
              teacher
   **hand out** = give (something) to this person,
                then to that person, then to
                another person, etc.
   **hang around/out (with)** = spend time relaxing
   **hang up** = (1) hang on a hanger or a hook
               (2) end a telephone conversation
   **have on** = wear
   **help out** = assist (someone)

K  **keep away (from)** = not give to
   **keep on** = continue

L  **lay off** = stop employment
   **leave on** = (1) not turn off (a light, a machine)
               (2) not take off (clothing)
   **look into** = investigate
   **look over** = examine carefully
   **look out (for)** = be careful
   **look up** = look for information in a dictionary,
               a telephone directory, an
               encyclopedia, etc.

P  **pay back** = return borrowed money to (someone)
   **pick up** = lift
   **point out** = call attention to

*(continued)*

**print out** = create a paper copy from a computer

**put away** = put (something) in its usual or proper place

**put back** = return (something) to its original place

**put down** = stop holding or carrying

**put off** = postpone

**put on** = put clothes on one's body

**put out** = extinguish (stop) a fire, a cigarette

R    **run into** = meet by chance

**run out (of)** = finish the supply of (something)

S    **set out (for)** = begin a trip

**shut off** = stop a machine or a light, turn off

**sign up (for)** = put one's name on a list

**show up** = come, appear

**sit around (with)** = sit and do nothing

**sit back** = put one's back against a chair back

**sit down** = go from standing to sitting

**speak up** = speak louder

**stand up** = go from sitting to standing

**start over** = begin again

**stay up** = not go to bed

T    **take back** = return

**take off** = (1) remove clothes from one's body (2) ascend in an airplane

**take out** = invite out and pay

**talk over** = discuss

**tear down** = destroy a building

**tear out (of)** = remove (paper) by tearing

**tear up** = tear into small pieces

**think over** = consider

**throw away/out** = put in the trash, discard

**try on** = put on clothing to see if it fits

**turn around**
**turn back** } change to the opposite direction

**turn down** = decrease the volume

**turn off** = stop a machine or a light

**turn on** = start a machine or a light

**turn over** = turn the top side to the bottom

**turn up** = increase the volume

W    **wake up** = stop sleeping

**watch out (for)** = be careful

**work out** = solve

**write down** = write a note on a piece of paper

# UNIT C: Prepositions

**NOTE:** See the *Fundamentals of English Grammar Workbook* appendix for practice exercises for preposition combinations.

## C-1 Preposition Combinations: Introduction

| | |
|---|---|
| ADJ + PREP<br>(a) Ali is *absent from* class today.<br><br>V + PREP<br>(b) This book *belongs to* me. | *At, from, of, on,* and *to* are examples of prepositions.<br>Prepositions are often combined with adjectives, as in (a), and verbs, as in (b). |

## C-2 Preposition Combinations: A Reference List

**A**
*be* absent from
*be* accustomed to
    add (*this*) to (*that*)
*be* acquainted with
    admire (*someone*) for (*something*)
*be* afraid of
    agree with (*someone*) about (*something*)
*be* angry at / with (*someone*) about / over (*something*)
    apologize to (*someone*) for (*something*)
    apply for (*something*)
    approve of
    argue with (*someone*) about / over (*something*)
    arrive at (*a building / a room*)
    arrive in (*a city / a country*)
    ask (*someone*) about (*something*)
    ask (*someone*) for (*something*)
*be* aware of

**B**
*be* bad for
    believe in
    belong to
*be* bored with / by
    borrow (*something*) from (*someone*)

**C**
*be* clear to
    combine with
    compare (*this*) to / with (*that*)
    complain to (*someone*) about (*something*)
*be* composed of
    concentrate on
    consist of
*be* crazy about
*be* crowded with
*be* curious about

**D**
    depend on (*someone*) for (*something*)
*be* dependent on (*someone*) for (*something*)

*be* devoted to
    die of / from
*be* different from
    disagree with (*someone*) about (*something*)
*be* disappointed in
    discuss (*something*) with (*someone*)
    divide (*this*) into (*that*)
*be* divorced from
*be* done with
    dream about / of
    dream of

**E**
*be* engaged to
*be* equal to
    escape from (*a place*)
*be* excited about
    excuse (*someone*) for (*something*)
    excuse from
*be* exhausted from

**F**
*be* familiar with
*be* famous for
    feel about
    feel like
    fill (*something*) with
*be* finished with
    forgive (*someone*) for (*something*)
*be* friendly to / with
*be* frightened of / by
*be* full of

**G**
    get rid of
*be* gone from
*be* good for
    graduate from

(continued)

**H**
happen to
*be* happy about (*something*)
*be* happy for (*someone*)
hear about / of (*something*) from (*someone*)
help (*someone*) with (*something*)
hide (*something*) from (*someone*)
hope for
*be* hungry for

**I**
insist on
*be* interested in
introduce (*someone*) to (*someone*)
invite (*someone*) to (*something*)
*be* involved in

**K**
*be* kind to
know about

**L**
laugh at
leave for (a *place*)
listen to
look at
look for
look forward to
look like

**M**
*be* made of
*be* married to
matter to
*be* the matter with
multiply (*this*) by (*that*)

**N**
*be* nervous about
*be* nice to

**O**
*be* opposed to

**P**
pay for
*be* patient with
*be* pleased with / about
play with
point at
*be* polite to
prefer (*this*) to (*that*)

*be* prepared for
protect (*this*) from (*that*)
*be* proud of
provide (*someone*) with

**Q**
*be* qualified for

**R**
read about
*be* ready for
*be* related to
rely on
*be* responsible for

**S**
*be* sad about
*be* satisfied with
*be* scared of / by
search for
separate (*this*) from (*that*)
*be* similar to
speak to / with (*someone*) about (*something*)
stare at
subtract (*this*) from (*that*)
*be* sure of / about

**T**
take care of
talk about (*something*)
talk to / with (*someone*) about (*something*)
tell (*someone*) about (*something*)
*be* terrified of / by
thank (*someone*) for (*something*)
think about / of
*be* thirsty for
*be* tired from
*be* tired of
translate from (*one language*) to (*another*)

**U**
*be* used to

**W**
wait for
wait on
warn about / of
wave at
wonder about
*be* worried about

# Listening Script

## Getting Started

### EXERCISE 1 ▶ p. xii.

**Part I**

*It's Nice to Meet You*

DANIEL: Hi. My name is Daniel.
SOFIA: Hi. I'm Sofia. It's nice to meet you.
DANIEL: Nice to meet you too. Where are you from?
SOFIA: I'm from Montreal. How about you?
DANIEL: I'm from Miami.
SOFIA: Are you a new student?
DANIEL: Yes, and no. This is my third year of college, but I'm new here.
SOFIA: This is my second year here. I'm in the business school. I really like it.
DANIEL: Oh, my major is economics! Maybe we'll have a class together. So, tell me a little more about yourself. What do you like to do in your free time?
SOFIA: I love the outdoors. I spend a lot of time in the mountains. I hike on weekends. I write about it on social media.
DANIEL: I spend a lot of time outdoors too. I like the beach. In the summer, I swim every day.
SOFIA: This town has a great beach.
DANIEL: Yeah, I want to go there! Now, when I introduce you to the group, I have to write your full name on the board. What's your last name, and how do you spell it?
SOFIA: It's Sanchez. S-A-N-C-H-E-Z.
DANIEL: My last name is Willson — with two "l"s: W-I-L-L-S-O-N.
SOFIA: Oh, it looks like our time is up. I enjoyed our conversation.
DANIEL: Thanks. I enjoyed it too.

## Chapter 8: Connecting Ideas: Punctuation and Meaning

### EXERCISE 11 ▶ p. 233.

*Paying It Forward*

A few days ago, a friend and I were driving from Benton Harbor to Chicago. We didn't have any delays for the first hour, but we ran into some highway construction near Chicago. The traffic wasn't moving. My friend and I sat and waited. We talked about our jobs, our families, and the terrible traffic. Slowly it started to move.

We noticed a black sports car on the shoulder. Its blinker was on. The driver obviously wanted to get back into traffic. Car after car passed without letting him in. I decided to do a good deed, so I motioned for him to get in line ahead of me. He waved thanks, and I waved back at him.

All the cars had to stop at a toll booth a short way down the road. I held out my money to pay my toll, but the toll-taker just smiled and waved me on. She told me that the man in the black sports car had already paid my toll. Wasn't that a nice way of saying thank you?

### EXERCISE 15 ▶ p. 235.

*A Strong Storm*

1. The noise lasted only a short time, but the wind and rain …
2. Some roads were under water, but ours …
3. Our neighbors didn't lose any trees, but we …
4. My son got scared, but my daughter …
5. My son couldn't sleep, but my daughter …
6. My daughter can sleep through anything, but my son …
7. We still need help cleaning up from the storm, but our neighbors …
8. We will be OK, but some people …

### EXERCISE 28 ▶ p. 243.

*Strange Allergies*

Allergies make people sneeze, cough, itch, or turn red. Common causes of allergies are dust, flower pollen, animal fur, and nuts. There are other things that cause allergies, but they are not so well known. Dark chocolate can make some people sneeze. The metal in cell phones can cause some people's skin to turn red and itch. Cold weather and leather clothing can also cause redness and itching in some people.

### EXERCISE 33 ▶ p. 246.

1. Even though I looked all over the house for my keys, …
2. Although it was a hot summer night, we went inside and shut the windows because …
3. My brother came to my graduation ceremony even though …
4. Because the package cost so much to send, …

5. Because gas is so expensive, …
6. Although the soccer team won the game, …

## Chapter 9: Comparisons

### EXERCISE 7 ▶ p. 254.

*Opinions*

1. Old shoes are more comfortable than new shoes.
2. Food from other countries is better than food from my country.
3. Winter is more enjoyable for me than summer.
4. Cooked vegetables are more delicious than raw vegetables.
5. Taking a bath is more relaxing than taking a shower.
6. Writing English is easier than speaking English.
7. Science is more interesting than history.
8. A math test is more stressful than an English test.

### EXERCISE 13 ▶ p. 257.

*My Family*

1. My brothers are shorter than my sisters.
2. My mother is the tallest person in our family.
3. My father is a fun person to be around. He seems happy all the time.
4. My grandmother was happier when she was younger.
5. I have twin brothers. They are older than me.
6. I have another brother. He is the funniest person in our family.
7. My sister is a doctor. She is a wise person.
8. My grandfather is also a doctor. He is the wisest person I know.

### EXERCISE 30 ▶ p. 267.

**Part II**
5. Tom has never told a funny joke.
6. Food has never tasted better.
7. I've never slept on a hard mattress.
8. I've never seen a scarier movie.

### EXERCISE 37 ▶ p. 271.

1. Frank owns a coffee shop. Business is busier this year for him than last year.
2. I've know Steven for years. He's the friendliest person I know.
3. Sam expected a hard test, but it wasn't as hard as he expected.
4. The road ends here. This is as far as we can go.
5. Jon's decision to leave his job was the worst decision he has ever made.
6. I don't know if we'll get to the theater on time, but I'm driving as fast as I can.
7. When you do the next assignment, please be more careful.
8. Is dinner ready? I've never been hungrier.
9. It takes about an hour to drive to the airport, and my flight takes an hour. So the drive takes as long as my flight.

### EXERCISE 41 ▶ p. 273.

1. a. A sidewalk is as wide as a road.
   b. A road is wider than a sidewalk.
2. a. A hill isn't as high as a mountain.
   b. A hill is higher than a mountain.
3. a. In general, hiking along a mountain path is more dangerous than climbing a mountain peak.
   b. In general, hiking along a mountain path is less dangerous than climbing a mountain peak.
4. a. Toes are longer than fingers.
   b. Fingers aren't as long as toes.
   c. Toes are shorter than fingers.
5. a. Basic math isn't as hard as algebra.
   b. Algebra is harder than basic math.
   c. Basic math is as confusing as algebra.
   d. Basic math is less confusing than algebra.

### EXERCISE 48 ▶ p. 277.

*Gold vs. Silver*

Gold is similar to silver. They are both valuable metals that people use for jewelry, but they aren't the same. Gold is not the same color as silver. Gold is also different from silver in cost: gold is more expensive than silver.

*Two Zebras*

Look at the two zebras in the picture. Their names are Zee and Bee. Zee looks like Bee. Is Zee exactly the same as Bee? The pattern of the stripes on each zebra in the world is unique. No two zebras are exactly alike. Even though Zee and Bee are similar to each other, they are different from each other in the exact pattern of their stripes.

## Chapter 10: The Passive

### EXERCISE 24 ▶ p. 294.

*A Bike Accident*

A: Did you hear about the accident outside the dorm entrance?
B: No. What happened?
A: A guy on a bike was hit by a taxi.
B: Was he injured?
A: Yeah. Someone called an ambulance. He was taken to City Hospital and treated in the emergency room for cuts and bruises.
B: What happened to the taxi driver?
A: He was arrested for reckless driving.
B: He's lucky that the bicyclist wasn't killed.

### EXERCISE 36 ▶ p. 301.

1. This fruit is spoiled. I think I'd better throw it out.
2. When we got to the post office, it was closed.
3. Oxford University is located in Oxford, England.
4. Haley doesn't like to ride in elevators. She's scared of small spaces.
5. What's the matter? Are you hurt?
6. Excuse me. Could you please tell me how to get to the bus station from here? I am lost.

7. Your name is Tom Hood? Are you related to Mary Hood?
8. Where's my wallet? It's gone! Did someone take it?
9. Oh, no! Look at my sunglasses. I sat on them, and now they are broken.
10. It's starting to rain. Are all of the windows shut?

## EXERCISE 40 ▶ p. 304.

1. Jane doesn't like school because of the boring classes and assignments.
2. The store manager stole money from the cash register. His shocked employees couldn't believe it.
3. I bought a new camera. I read the directions twice, but I didn't understand them. They were too confusing for me.
4. I was out to dinner with a friend and spilled a glass of water on his pants. I felt very embarrassed, but he was very nice about it.
5. Every year for their anniversary, I surprise my parents with dinner at a different restaurant.
6. We didn't enjoy the movie. It was too scary for the kids.

## EXERCISE 45 ▶ p. 306.

1. In winter, the weather gets …
2. In summer, the weather gets …
3. I think I'll stop working. I'm getting …
4. My brother is losing some of his hair. He's getting …
5. Could I have a glass of water? I'm getting really …
6. You don't look well. Are you getting …

## Chapter 11: Count/Noncount Nouns and Articles

## EXERCISE 11 ▶ p. 321.

1. At our school, teachers don't use chalk anymore.
2. Where is the soap? Did you use all of it?
3. The manager's suggestions were very helpful.
4. Which suggestion sounded best to you?
5. Is this ring made of real gold?
6. We have a lot of storms with thunder and lightning.
7. During the last storm, I found my daughter under her bed.
8. Please put the cap back on the toothpaste.
9. What do you want to do with all this stuff in the hall closet?
10. We have too much soccer and hockey equipment.

## EXERCISE 31 ▶ p. 332.

1. We have a holiday next week.
2. What are you going to (*gonna*) do?
3. I don't know. Do you have a suggestion?
4. Let's go shopping at the new mall.
5. They're having a big sale.
6. Actually, I'm going there in an hour.
7. Do you want to (*wanna*) come?
8. I can't. I just got a message.
9. I need to call my boss.
10. Hmmm. That's unusual. He's on vacation.

## EXERCISE 39 ▶ p. 336.

*Ice-Cream Headaches*

Have you ever eaten something really cold like ice cream and suddenly gotten a headache? This is known as an "ice-cream headache." About 30 percent of the population gets this type of headache. Here is one theory about why ice-cream headaches occur. The roof of your mouth has a lot of nerves. When something cold touches these nerves, they want to warm up your brain. Your blood vessels swell up, and this causes pain. Ice-cream headaches generally go away after about 30–60 seconds. The best way to avoid these headaches is to keep cold food off the roof of your mouth.

## Chapter 12: Adjective Clauses

## EXERCISE 23 ▶ p. 356.

*My Mother's Hospital Stay*

1. The doctor who my mother saw first spent a lot of time with her.
2. The doctor I called for a second opinion was very patient and understanding.
3. The room that my mother had was private.
4. The medicine which she took worked better than she expected.
5. The hospital that my mom chose specializes in women's care.
6. The day my mom came home happened to be her birthday.
7. I thanked the people that helped my mom.
8. The staff whom I met were all excellent.

## EXERCISE 32 ▶ p. 361.

1. The plane which I'm taking to Denver leaves at 7:00 a.m.
2. The store that has the best vegetables is also the most expensive.
3. The eggs my husband made me for breakfast were cold.
4. The person who sent me an email was trying to get my bank account number.
5. The hotel clerk my wife spoke with on the phone said he would give us a room with a view.

## EXERCISE 37 ▶ p. 364.

1. I like the people whose house we went to.
2. The man whose daughter is a doctor is very proud.
3. The man who's standing by the window has a daughter at Oxford University.
4. I know a girl whose parents are both airline pilots.
5. I know a girl who's lonely because her parents travel a lot.
6. I met a 70-year-old woman who's planning to go to college.

## EXERCISE 40 ▶ p. 365.

*Friendly Advice*

A: A magazine that I saw at the doctor's office had an article you ought to read. It's about the importance of exercise in dealing with stress.

B: Why do you think I should read an article which deals with exercise and stress?

A: If you stop and think for a minute, you can answer that question yourself. You're under a lot of stress, and you don't get any exercise.

B: The stress that I have at work doesn't bother me. It's just a normal part of my job. And I don't have time to exercise.

A: Well, you should make time. Anyone whose job is as stressful as yours should make physical exercise part of their daily routine.

## Chapter 13: Gerunds and Infinitives

## EXERCISE 4 ▶ p. 371.

1. A: Do you have any plans for this weekend?
   B: Henry and I talked about seeing the dinosaur exhibit at the museum.
2. A: When you finish doing your homework, could you help me in the kitchen?
   B: Sure.
3. A: I didn't understand the answer. Would you mind explaining it?
   B: I'd be happy to.
4. A: I'm thinking about not attending the meeting tomorrow.
   B: Really? Why? I hope you go. We need your input.
5. A: I've been working on this math problem for an hour, and I still don't understand it.
   B: Well, don't give up. Keep trying.

## EXERCISE 23 ▶ p. 382.

A: Have you made any vacation plans?
B: Kind of. We're going to take a staycation.
A: You mean you're going to stay home and vacation?
B: Yeah. To be honest, I don't like traveling so much. I hate flying. It's so uncomfortable nowadays.
A: But your wife loves to travel, doesn't she?

B: Right. But we don't see our kids so much because they're in college. So we decided to spend time here so we can see them, and we can be tourists in our own town.
A: So, what are you planning to see?
B: Well, we haven't seen the new Museum of Space yet. There's also a new art exhibit downtown. And my wife would like to go sailing in the harbor. Actually, when we began talking about it, we discovered there were lots of things to do.
A: Sounds like a great solution!
B: Yeah, we're both really excited about seeing our kids and more of our own town.

## Chapter 14: Noun Clauses

## EXERCISE 22 ▶ p. 412.

1. WOMAN: My English teacher is really good. I like her a lot.
   MAN: That's great! I'm glad you're enjoying your class.
2. MOM: How do you feel, honey? You might have the flu.
   SON: I'm OK, Mom. Honest. I don't have the flu.
3. MAN: Did you really fail your chemistry course? How is that possible?
   WOMAN: I didn't study hard enough. Now I won't be able to graduate on time.
4. MAN: Rachel! Hello! It's nice to see you.
   WOMAN: Hi, it's nice to be here. Thank you for inviting me.
5. WOMAN: Carol has left. Look. Her closet is empty. Her suitcases are gone. She won't be back. I just know it!
   MAN: She'll be back.

## EXERCISE 40 ▶ p. 424.

Angela called and asked me where Bill was. I told her he was in the lunchroom. She asked when he would be back. I said he would be back around 2:00. I asked her if I could do something for her.

She said that Bill had the information she needed, and only he could help her. I told her that I would leave him a message. She thanked me and hung up.

# Trivia Answers

## Chapter 9, Exercise 4, p. 252.

1. larger       T
2. colder       T
3. bigger       F [Asia is bigger than Africa.]
4. hotter       T
5. wetter       T
6. deeper       F [The Pacific Ocean is deeper than the Atlantic Ocean.]
7. more humid       T
8. more crowded       F [China is more crowded than Canada.]
9. longer       T
10. higher       F [The Himalayas are higher than the Andes.]

## Chapter 9, Exercise 10, p. 256.

2. The coldest ocean is the Arctic. / The Arctic is the coldest ocean.
3. The biggest ocean is the Pacific. / The Pacific is the biggest ocean.
4. The windiest continent is Antarctica. / Antarctica is the windiest continent.
5. The hottest continent is Africa. / Africa is the hottest continent.
6. The most populated continent is Asia. / Asia is the most populated continent.
7. The largest country in Asia is China. / China is the largest country in Asia.
8. The smallest country in Asia is the Maldives. / The Maldives is the smallest country in Asia.
9. The tallest mountain is Denali. / Denali is the tallest mountain.
10. The lowest mountain is Mount Fuji. / Mount Fuji is the lowest mountain.
11. The heaviest animal is the whale. / The whale is the heaviest animal.
12. The fastest animal is the cheetah. / The cheetah is the fastest animal.

## Chapter 9, Exercise 42, p. 273.

Seattle and Singapore have more rain than Manila in December.
[Manila: 58 mm. or 2.3 in.; Seattle: 161 mm. or 6.3 in.; Singapore: 306 mm. or 12 in.]

## Chapter 9, Exercise 44, p. 275.

2. Indonesia has more volcanoes than Japan.
3. Saturn has more moons than Venus.
4. Saõ Paulo, Brazil, has more people than New York City.
5. Finland has more islands than Greece.
6. Nepal has more mountains than Switzerland.
7. A banana has more sugar than an apple.
8. The dark meat of a chicken has more fat than the white meat of a chicken.

## Chapter 10, Exercise 18, p. 291.

3. a. Princess Dianna was killed in a car crash in 1997.
4. j. Marie and Pierre Curie discovered radium.
5. f. Oil was discovered in Saudi Arabia in 1938.
6. i. Nelson Mandela was released from prison in 1990.
7. b. Michael Jackson died in 2009.
8. d. Leonardo da Vinci painted the *Mona Lisa*.
9. e. John F. Kennedy was elected president of the United States in 1960.
10. g. Romeo and Juliet were kept apart by their parents.

## Chapter 10, Exercise 29, p. 298.

1. sand
2. whales
3. China and Mongolia
4. small spaces

## Chapter 11, Exercise 42, p. 338.

1. Ø ... Ø       T
2. The ... Ø       T
3. Ø ... Ø       F [Austria]
4. The ... Ø       T
5. The ... the       F
6. The ... Ø ... the       T
7. Ø       F [psychology / psychiatry]
8. Ø ... Ø       T [It also lies in Uganda and borders Kenya.]
9. Ø ... the       T
10. The       F [The Himalayas]

# Index

| | |
|---|---|
| Capitalization, 229, 230, 416<br>   (*Look on page 229 and also on pages 339 and 416.*) | The numbers following the words listed in the index refer to page numbers in the text. |
| ***By hand,*** 383*fn.*<br>   (*Look at the footnote on page 383.*) | The letters *fn.* mean "footnote." Footnotes are at the bottom of a chart or the bottom of a page. |

# Credits

**Photo Credits:** Page **xii**: Mjth/Shutterstock; **228**: Markus Mainka/Shutterstock; **229**: Laurent davoust/123RF; **230** (all images): Marina113/123RF; **231**: Lightspring/Shutterstock; **232** (top): Thamkc/123RF; **232** (bottom): Arena Creative/Shutterstock; **233** (tarantula): Mirek Kijewski/Shutterstock; **233** (elephants): Claudia Paulussen/Shutterstock; **233** (dolphin): Christian Musat/Shutterstock; **233** (toll booth): S-F/Shutterstock; **235**: Samuel Acosta/Shutterstock; **238**: Markus Pfaff/Shutterstock; **241**: Larry Rains/123RF; **242**: G215/123RF; **243**: Alex Cofaru/Shutterstock; **244**: Xray Computer/Shutterstock; **245** (top): Ollyy/Shutterstock; **245** (bottom): Feruz Malik/Shutterstock; **247** (writing with pen): Sakkmesterke/Shutterstock; **247** (baseball): Gino Santa Maria/Shutterstock; **248**: Jordan Tan/Shutterstock; **250**: Murali Nath/123RF; **250** (Daniel): Wang Tom/123RF; **250** (Taka): Arek_malang/Shutterstock; **252**: Almoond/123RF; **253**: John McLaird/123RF; **256**: Ildogesto/Shuttertsock; **257**: Dolgachov/123RF; **261** (diamond): Alexander Maslennikov/Shutterstock; **261** (Great Wall): Songquan Deng/Shutterstock; **261** (volcano): Orxy/Shutterstock; **263** (top): Stefanolunardi/Shutterstock; **263** (bottom): Sergey Novikov/Shutterstock; **265** (boy & balloon): Sabphoto/123RF; **265** (ambulance): Cheryl Casey/Shutterstock; **265** (globe): Serg64/Shutterstock; **267**: Serazetdinov/Shutterstock; **268** (Niki): Bruno135/123RF; **268** (Alex): Rido/123RF; **268** (Emilio): Auremar/123RF; **268** (Maya): 123RF; **270** (Tia): Sjenner13/123RF; **270** (Amira): Antonio Guillem/123RF; **270** (Jasmine): Michel Borges/Shutterstock; **270** (Sachi): Kenneth Man/Shutterstock; **270** (Emily): Jon Barlow/Pearson Education Ltd; **271** (ox): Prapass/Shutterstock; **271** (mule): Robynrg/Shutterstock; **271** (hornet): Melinda Fawver/123RF; **273**: Thomas Dutour/123RF; **274**: Sam D Cruz/123RF; **276** (geese): E. O./Shutterstock; **276** (duck): Anatolii Tsekhmister/123RF; **277** (orange): Roman Samokhin/Shutterstock; **277** (peach): Natika/123RF; **277** (silver & gold): Konstantin Inozemtcev/123RF; **278**: apoplexia/RF123; **279**: Anek Suwannaphoom/123RF; **280**: Andreas G. Karelias/Shutterstock; **284**: Sergey Mironov/Shutterstock; **285**: Oleksiy Mark/Shutterstock; **286**: Noviantoko Tri Arijanto/123RF; **287**: Elena Dijour/Shutterstock; **288**: Peshkova/Shutterstock; **289**: Action Sports Photography/Shutterstock; **291**: Wdg Photo/Shutterstock; **292**: Travelview/Shutterstock; **293**: Bea Rue/Shutterstock; **294** (police officer): Paul Vasarhelyi/123RF; **294** (bicyclist): Szefei/Shutterstock; **295**: Alberto cervantes/Shutterstock; **296**: Karelnoppe/Shutterstock; **297**: Africa Studio/Shutterstock; **299** (anxious man): Kurhan/Shutterstock; **299** (confident woman): Iodrakon/Shutterstock; **302** (shark): Clay S. Turner/Shutterstock; **302** (swimmer): Pacter Gudella/123RF; **303** (top left): Neil Lang/Shutterstock; **303** (top right): Jacob Lund/Shutterstock; **303** (bottom): Kittipong Jirasukhanont/123RF; **304**: Vladimir Tarasov/123RF; **306**: Mark Bowden/123RF; **309**: Rawpixel.com/Shutterstock; **310**: Fejas/Shutterstock; **312**: Rob Wilson/Shutterstock; **313**: Nick Reynolds Photography/Shutterstock; **315**: Poznyakov/Shutterstock; **316**: Robyn Mackenzie/Shutterstock; **317** (blue chair): Photobac/Shutterstock; **317** (red chair): Photosync/Shutterstock; **317** (orange chair): Aleksandr Kurganov/Shutterstock; **322**: DOPhoto/Shutterstock; **325** (eye glasses): Aimy27feb/123RF; **325** (broken window): Maroon Studio/Shutterstock; **325** (drinking glass): Belchonock/123RF; **326** (brown chicken): Stockphoto mania/Shutterstock; **326** (chick): Anneka/Shutterstock; **326** (roast chicken): Dani Vincek/Shutterstock; **326** (fried chicken): Bigacis/Shutterstock; **326** (white chickens): Malcolm Harris/Pearson Education Ltd; **326** (free range chicken): Elenathewise/123RF; **327**: Miroslav Pesek/123RF; **328** (pasta with sauce): Subbotina/123RF; **328** (shopping basket): Cherries/Shutterstock; **329** (one dog): Wasitt Hemwarapornchai/Shutterstock; **329** (three dogs): Rybaltovskaya Marina/123RF; **330** (red house): Pixel Embargo/Shutterstock; **330** (ice cream scoop): Olga Lyubkina/Shutterstock; **330** (ice cream bowl): M. Unal Ozmen/Shutterstock; **333** (prisoner): Liron Peer/Shutterstock; **333** (bottom): Peter Engstrom/123RF; **334**: Sari ONeal/Shutterstock; **335**: Africa Studio/Shutterstock;

336 (center): Primagefactory/123RF; 336 (bottom): kastianz/Shutterstock; 337: Aetherial Images/Shutterstock; 338: Scanrail/123RF; 341: Tinseltown/Shutterstock; 342: Olga Khelmitskaya/123RF; 344: Andrey Armyagov/ Shutterstock; 345: Chris Noble/123RF; 346: Wavebreak Media Ltd/123RF; 347 (top): 3quarks/123RF; 347 (bottom): Budimir Jevtic/Shutterstock; 348: Rido/Shutterstock; 349: Suzanne Tucker/Shutterstock; 350: Alexander Raths/Shutterstock; 351 (top): Kasto/123RF; 351 (bottom): Katarzyna Białasiewicz/123RF; 352: Eric Isselee/123RF; 353: Sirinapa/123RF; 354 (like symbol): Umarazak/Shutterstock; 355: Flamingo Images/Shutterstock; 356: Mark Bowden/123RF; 357: V_E/Shutterstock; 361: Ljansempoi/Shutterstock; 362: Michaeljung/Shutterstock; 363: Shutterstock; 365: Focus and Blur/Shutterstock; 368: Anna Shepulova/ Shutterstock; 369: Federico Rostagno/Shutterstock; 370 (bakery owners): Racorn/123RF; 370 (eating hamburger): Peter Albrektsen/Shutterstock; 370 (stressed woman): Voyagerix/Shutterstock; 371: Chitsanupong Chuenthananont/123RF; 372: Olga Khoroshunova/123RF; 373 (skier): Shutterstock; 373 (camping): Bozulek/Shutterstock; 373 (bowling): Africa Studio/Shutterstock; 373 (ice skating): Roman Babakin/ Shutterstock; 373 (sailing): Ivan Smuk/Shutterstock; 373 (hiking): Maridav/Shutterstock; 373 (fishing): Mark Bowden/123RF; 373 (jogging): Fotokostic/Shutterstock; 373 (swimming): Jane September/Shutterstock; 373 (shopping): Zoriana Zaitseva/Shutterstock; 375: Belchonock/123RF; 377 (top right): Anastasia Vish/123RF; 377 (bottom): Wang Tom/123RF; 380 (woman): Kinga/Shutterstock; Aaron Amat/Shutterstock; 382: Alexei Novikov/123RF; 385 (scissors): Tsz-shan Kwok/Pearson Education Asia Ltd; 385 (thermometer): Kanchana Phikulthong/123RF; 385 (needle & thread): Konstantin Kirillov/123RF; 385 (broom): Jarp5/123RF; 385 (spoon) Pirtuss/Shutterstock; 385 (hammer): Sergiy Kuzmin/Shutterstock; 385 (shovel): Lostintrance/ Shutterstock; 385 (saw): Gearstd/Shutterstock; 386: Rido/123RF; 387: Mark Brooks/123RF; 388: Wavebreak Media Ltd/123RF; 389: Wang Tom/123RF; 390: Mangostock/Shutterstock; 391: Mangostock/Shutterstock; 393 (top): Joao Virissimo/Shutterstock; 393 (bottom): Zapp2Photo/Shutterstock; 394: Gleb TV/123RF; 395 (top): Angela Waye/123RF; 395 (center): ChristianChan/Shutterstock; 398: Rob Marmion/123RF; 400: Voin_Sveta/ Shutterstock; 402: Michaeljung/Shutterstock; 404: Oleksiy Mark/Shutterstock; 407: Goodluz/123RF; 408: Ion Chiosea/123RF; 409: Dolgachov/123RF; 410: Rawpixel/123RF; 411 (capsule): Nirot Sriprasit/123RF; 411 (party): Wavebreakmedia/Shutterstock; 412: Nicoelnino/Shutterstock; 413: Olena Yakobchuk/Shutterstock; 414: Andriy Popov/123RF; 415: Elwynn/Shutterstock; 416: Petr Podrouzek/123RF; 417: Andreypopov/123RF; 418 (top): Jon Barlow/Pearson Education Ltd; 418 (bottom right): StockLite/Shutterstock; 421: Vadim Guzhva/123RF; 422: Ilic Nikola/123RF; 424: Katja Heinemann/Cavan/Aurora Photos/Alamy Stock Photo; 429: Igors Rusakovs/123RF.

**Illustration credits:** Don Martinetti—**236, 237, 254, 268, 269, 277, 282, 283, 426**

# NOTES